THE POWER OF 4™

Health, Vitality, Longevity and Fat Loss

THE
POWER
OF 4™

Your ultimate guide guaranteed
to change your body and
transform your life

PAULA OWENS

Copyright © 2008 by Paula Owens

ISBN: 978-0-615-25750-1

Printed In the United States of America

CONTENTS

CHAPTER THREE

THE POWER OF LIFESTYLE

CHAPTER FOUR

ACKNOWLEDGEMENTS

I would be remiss not to acknowledge the value and knowledge I attained from these brilliant men: world-renowned Olympic strength coach, Charles Poliquin, Doctor Harry O. Eidenier, Jr., Ph.D. and Doctor Eric Serrano, M.D.

Love to my Mother for instilling within me her philosophy of the four "Ds" – drive, dedication, determination and desire.

My heartfelt thanks and love to friends, Laura Kobar and Margaret Ott, for their support and time spent proof reading my manuscript.

I wish to express gratitude and love to my faithful clientele, as well as all of my wonderful, amazing friends who have supported me throughout this process.

Last but not least, I thank you for reading *THE POWER OF 4*. I believe all of us are entitled to a life of balance and health on all levels: physically, emotionally, intellectually, mentally and spiritually. It is there for all of us if we so desire. My passion thrives as I continue my journey evolving. My intention and purpose is to inspire and empower every one of you – to share my philosophy and knowledge in order to transform the lives of others.

Paula Owens

FOREWORD

By Harry Eidenier, Jr., Ph.D.

As a doctor involved in the area of alternative medicine, I find *THE POWER OF 4* to be the absolute best I've seen on the subject of nutrition, supplementation and exercise in the past thirty years.

Perhaps the most remarkable thing about Paula's book is that it took so long for someone to transpire all of this information to share with the public. Expert information defines *THE POWER OF 4*. There is no question that Ms. Owens is an expert in her field that combines nutrition, lifestyle, exercise and supplementation. This information has been needed for at least thirty years that I know of.

At the time Ms. Owens asked me to write the foreword, I had already admired her expertise in the area of exercise physiology, supplemental feeding and diet management. *THE POWER OF 4* combines her expertise and experience together and provides a comprehensive, well organized, easy to understand book that will allow the reader to improve themselves or help their clients in many ways.

Further, I sincerely believe that this book should be used as a text in any institution of higher learning where the student is pursuing a degree in nutrition, exercise physiology or dietetics.

It is full of useful information for both the lay person and the professional.

After my thirty-two years as a Ph.D. in the field of alternative medicine, I was able to glean a world of useful information on supplementation, diet and exercise. If you are at all interested in holistic nutrition information, correct supplementation and how to exercise to really help yourself or your client, this is a must read. *THE POWER OF 4* is the absolute best!

Harry O. Eidenier, Jr., Ph.D.

FOREWORD

By Charles Poliquin

During my last thirty years as a strength coach and educator, I have come across many brilliant students, one of them being Paula Owens.

Paula's book, **THE POWER OF 4**, is a gift of knowledge on life improvement. That collection of health and lifestyle wisdom tips is a direct reflection of her soul and intentions – precise, direct, pensive, thoughtful, and of course, always very kind and loving.

I have known Paula for over fifteen years as a student, then as a colleague. She genuinely is a person who brings the best out of everyone she meets.

The greatest assets of **THE POWER OF 4** are that Paula presents countless gems that all do work. No waste, no excess verbiage –just the absolute best – like Paula.

Charles Poliquin
Olympic Strength Coach
www.charlespoliquin.com

INTRODUCTION

THE POWER OF 4 was written specifically for you. Do you want to change your body? Lose weight? Increase your energy? Transform your life? Do you want to find out what it takes to achieve optimal *Health, Vitality, Longevity and Fat Loss*? What if I told you that *THE POWER OF 4* guarantees healthy fat loss and complete physique transformation?

THE POWER OF 4 has come from my thirty years of experience as a personal fitness expert and holistic nutritionist. My intention is to share with you what works and what does not. I have had the pleasure of helping people attain health naturally, completely transforming their physiques by implementing *THE POWER OF 4*. The four 'POWERS' include nutrition, lifestyle, exercise and proper supplementation.

I am delighted, blessed and very grateful for the opportunity to present my book to you. My extensive studies throughout the years have provided me with an abundance of knowledge and vast experience. My purpose for writing this book is to reveal that information and my philosophy to you. The result? An empowered, inspired you, living a healthy life full of vitality and balance with a body you'll love as you implement *THE POWER OF 4.*

CHAPTER 1-1

WHAT IS HOLISTIC HEALTH?

"A wise man should consider that health is the greatest of human blessings."
~Hippocrates

If you're like most people you've tried one diet after another, you've read all of the latest books on losing weight, you engage in an exercise program and still haven't achieved the results you desire. Maybe you've taken steps to improve your health; however you'd like to further enhance your success. You will achieve higher levels of *Health, Vitality, Longevity and Fat Loss* from the *Winning Formulas* presented in *THE POWER OF 4.*

THE POWER OF 4 will expose you to the truth and what it takes to experience *Health, Vitality, Longevity and Fat Loss* so you can live a quality life and feel and look incredible!

Ask yourself these questions:

- Are you ready to invest in your most valuable asset – YOU?
- Are you sick and tired of feeling sick and tired?
- Do you want a lean, healthy body without dieting and depriving yourself?

- Do you want to experience a meaningful, joy-filled life?
- Do you want to experience improvements in your health and fitness?
- Do you want to live longer and enjoy all the gifts in your life? (Family, friends, nature, inner peace, community service, etc.)
- Do you want to overcome chronic pain, heal your body and free yourself of toxic pharmaceutical medications?

Well, here you go! You will be forever transformed as you read **THE POWER OF 4** – *Your ultimate guide guaranteed to change your body and transform your life.*

People of all ages are concerned about their health, how they feel and how they look, disease prevention, as well as quality of life. Unfortunately, the majority of you have been brainwashed to believe in the concept of eating less fat, consuming fewer calories, undergoing cosmetic surgery and excessive exercise to attain **Health, Vitality, Longevity and Fat Loss.** How can you achieve complete wellness, naturally without gimmicks and artificial fixes? My **Winning Formulas for Health, Vitality, Longevity and Fat Loss** are a holistic approach which integrates all aspects of wellness encompassing body, mind, emotions, environment, community and spiritual health.

Holistic health is a "lifestyle" that requires you to be an active participant **taking control and responsibility** of various aspects of your life such as:

- A sensible exercise program
- Eating wholesome, organic foods
- Emotional and mental well-being
- Hormonal balance
- Optimal digestion
- Peace of mind and happiness
- Positive thoughts
- Restful sleep
- Quality relationships
- Spiritual connection and awareness
- Stress management, relaxation, meditation and breathing

Holistic health is a natural express and harmony of life. It consists of peace of mind, happiness and complete well-being on all levels – physical, emotional, intellectual, mental and spiritual. It is a balance, evolution and integration of these aspects. You are made up of spirit, mind and body. If there is a problem in one of these areas, it will affect the others as well.

Holistic health addresses the entire person and their current lifestyle. It focuses on prevention, health maintenance, high-level wellness and longevity. You are an active participant in the healing process of your life.

Holistic health is not portrayed by the individual you see in a magazine ad or on television with a bronzed tan, a chiseled six-pack abdomen, nibbling on lettuce and chicken breast. Nor is it the person you see at the gym spending countless hours on the elliptical trainer, botox injections, the latest celebrity diet craze or the individual who jogs twenty-five miles per week.

The truth is that no amount of exercise or cosmetic surgery will reshape your physique without attention to your lifestyle, deep-rooted emotions and nutrition. Most diets set you up to fail. They work against your natural biochemistry and program your body to store fat.

The sound nutrition, lifestyle, exercise and supplement principles found here in *THE POWER OF 4* will accelerate and heal your metabolism.

Implementing the information from *THE POWER OF 4* will generate an ideal, healthy weight and total well-being. Diets and weight loss gimmicks lead to a damaged metabolism. People who maintain their natural weight range usually have a healthy relationship with food, viewing it as nourishment. They enjoy food and eating without feelings of guilt, anxiety or obsession.

The American population has been misinformed regarding what it takes to lose weight, attain the ultimate physique and live a healthy lifestyle.

Unfortunately, medical schools teach upcoming doctors little, if any, about nutrition or prevention of disease. Instead, doctors are taught how to prescribe toxic pharmaceutical drugs, making doctors the third leading cause of death. Most people seeking medical attention from an allopathic, conventional physician walk away thinking prescription drugs are the answer to everything. If the drug doesn't work, a larger dose is recommended, another drug is prescribed or the patient is blamed. There is seldom any mention of the natural alternatives or lifestyle changes. In the meantime, the underlying condition that prompted the visit in the first place is still there. It may be masked, but drugs cannot make it go away. After a period of time, it worsens or reappears in another form. Each patent medicine has a list of side effects that often make matters worse. Eventually, more drugs are needed to deal with them. This down-hill run leads to premature death.

A key component of wellness is self-acceptance. Many people use personal symptoms as excuses for a lack of initiative and sub-standard performance. Some individuals may feel that certain ailments are predetermined and identify themselves with their disease. Many believe that at age forty their mind, sight, hearing, libido, joints and physique are on the decline and degeneration is bound to happen. Even worse, society has become dependent upon pharmaceuticals, stimulants or processed foods for maintenance of the most basic human functions.

Sugar and other artificial stimulants are used for false energy production. In reality these deplete you of energy, wreak havoc on your health and leave you more exhausted on deeper levels.

Laxatives and diuretics are prescribed to purge the colon and bladder. Fertility drugs are available to help us reproduce. Alcohol and recreational drugs are abused in hopes of attaining a higher level of consciousness.

Consciousness is the product of brain activity, self-awareness and inner-life. It's the way you get in sync with yourself, connecting with who you are on a deeper level. Consciousness is the connection to your inner-self.

Individuals with a higher level of consciousness were found to have a reduced risk of developing Alzheimer's disease. Higher levels of consciousness can be achieved naturally through practices of meditation, prayer and spiritual evolution.

Your choice to read *THE POWER OF 4* is no accident. You will discover *Winning Formulas for Health, Vitality, Longevity and Fat Loss* from the inside out. Undeniable results are inevitable when you implement *THE POWER OF 4* which includes:

- The Power of Nutrition
- The Power of Lifestyle
- The Power of Physical Exercise
- The Power of Supplementation

The emphasis of *THE POWER OF 4*

- Alter body composition – lose fat and increase muscle
- Balance your adrenals, thyroid and sex hormones
- Effective stress management and breathing practices
- Eliminate your chances of metabolic syndrome (high blood pressure, elevated triglycerides and low HDL, increased inflammatory markers, abnormal insulin levels and obesity)
- Healthy functioning liver, gallbladder, kidney and bladder
- Ideal hydration
- Knowledge of supplementation
- Optimal digestion and healthy bowel/gut function
- Plenty of restful and quality sleep
- Proper balance of essential fatty acids
- Recovery and healing modalities
- Removal of harmful toxins and allergens
- Sensible exercise for fat loss versus fat acceleration
- Spiritual awareness and harmony
- Stabilized blood sugar
- Strong immune system
- Wholesome diet of quality foods including protein, carbohydrates and fats for optimal nourishment

Be mindful

Many of us operate in a robotic, autopilot manner throughout the day. Be aware of your thoughts and actions. This awareness creates a positive, unbelievable transformation.

Your subconscious belief system is very powerful. It generates your perceptions and feelings about life.

You radiate whatever level of consciousness you are currently feeling. And your body is the key to all this because you hold your emotions in your body. That is scientifically proven by none other than a great woman scientist, Candace Pert who says, "If you truly want to understand what's happening in your subconscious, look at your physical body. The body is where unresolved emotions and mental patterns accumulate." When you release emotions that no longer serve you, you release toxins from your body.

Your physical body is carved and created from your subconscious thoughts and feelings. Unhealthy, negative thoughts may manifest as excess weight, chronic aches and pains, elevated blood pressure or an autoimmune disease. Changing your thinking can alter your brain's neurochemistry. Positive emotional states are linked to prolonged life expectancy.

Read and reflect on the following information.

- Anti-depressants are used by 118 million individuals in the United States. Ninety million would not need these drugs if they would incorporate a balanced protocol of amino acid therapy in their healing regimen.

- Ninety percent of all individuals carry one or more parasites.

- Ninety percent of all diseases (cancer, diabetes, cardiovascular, depression, etc.) are easily prevented through proper nutrition, appropriate exercise, lifestyle modifications and adequate sunlight. None of these are ever promoted because the financial gain is minimal or nonexistent.

- Seven out of ten American adults are overweight or obese.

- The average American consumes an average of twenty pounds of additives, preservatives and colorings annually.

- The majority of the American population lead sedentary lives void of movement throughout the day; sitting at computers, watching television, playing videos games and enduring long commutes in our vehicles.

- The three top drugs prescribed in the United States, as stated by Dr. Eric Serrano, MD, are "Prilosec, amoxicillin (an antibiotic) and anti-depressants."

- The typical person consumes 150 pounds of sugar per year.

- The United States has a population with the most obese, sick and pharmaceutically medicated individuals.
- We eat meat from animals that feed on corn and soy-meal versus grass and pasture feeding. These animals are injected with antibiotics, synthetic estrogens and growth hormones.
- The media is controlled by Big Pharma, which spends billions every year to pay for article placement in big news sources like CNN, *USA Today* and New York Times.
- We live with a huge amount of stress and anxiety. We experience depression.

When one considers that there have been profound advances in nutrition, healthcare and medicine it is quite obvious that something has gone astray in our attempt to achieve practical and holistic health.

Now that you've been introduced to a small sample of the obstacles which derail us from living healthy and vibrant lives, ask yourself: "Who's the sole person responsible for taking control of my health, making the right decisions for me, creating healthier thought patterns and following through with action?"

Be Informed. Be Inspired. Be Empowered.

Allow **THE POWER OF 4** to change your body and transform your life starting now!

CHAPTER 1-2
GOAL SETTING – BE the Change

"Whatever you focus on you create more of. Whatever you believe, think and speak about yourself you create as your experience.
Whatever you flow emotional energy to you manifest in abundance."
~Carol Tuttle

Change begins with a thought. Change and transformation require energy. Creating outer change involves inner change at the mental and emotional level of your being. According to William James, M.D., often referred to as the father of American Psychology, "it takes twenty-one days to create a habit or permanent change."

Positive change always leads to sustainable gains in well-being and healing – emotionally, spiritually and physically.

Remember, there is always a period of inner work before evolving. The greater the outer change you wish to manifest, the greater the inner change that must be made first. Serious intention and desire to evolve requires emotional motivation. 'BE' that thought, 'DO' that action and you will 'HAVE' inevitable transformation.

Focus on your intention. An intention is a subtle energy that attracts what you want. It's a decision within that transforms your goal into reality. Your decision to change starts with a thought. Therein, behavioral change takes place. You are more likely to change your behavior by focusing on your intention.

Identify any obstacles to obtaining your goals. Visualize yourself following through with your goal, so that success is not only possible, it's inevitable. For example, you might decide in advance that every time you're tempted to eat ice cream after dinner, you will take a twenty minute walk or a hot bath instead. When this craving arises, it's a signal to take a walk or bath, not eat the ice cream.

My experience for success has been to keep it simple. Small, incremental changes over time result into life-altering rewards that are absolutely profound and definitely worth your efforts. Share and communicate your plan of action and goals with others such as friends, co-workers and family. Doing so reinforces your commitment to attain your goal. Focus on the positive reward of a behavior rather than the sacrifice or effort. Always plan to succeed.

In chapters two through five you will find the *Winning Formulas*. These are examples of specific goals. Focus on two *Winning Formulas* each and every week to strengthen your intention to create a leaner, healthier you from the inside out.

According to the Positive Psychology Center, writing about life goals is associated with enhanced well-being.

Write your two *Winning Formulas* down each and every week. Keep them in sight. Read them numerous times per day.

Locations you can place your *Winning Formulas*:

- Above the kitchen sink
- At the computer monitor
- At the telephone
- At your desk
- In your briefcase
- In your wallet
- Inside the medicine cabinet
- On the closet door
- On the dashboard of your vehicle
- On the front door
- On your mirror
- On the refrigerator

Retain your vision of these two weekly *Winning Formulas* in your thought process. What you concentrate on expands. You do not have to know how. Consciously keep the vision of what you aspire to at the forefront of your mind. Think about what you want instead of what you do not want. Declare your goals. Give them life. Believe in yourself. Get excited. Reach beyond. Expect the best!

With the information from *THE POWER OF 4* plus your drive, desire, dedication and determination you will achieve optimal health, inner peace and physique transformation. Guaranteed!

The time is now! Take control and responsibility for yourself. Your choices made today greatly impact and influence your state of balance and health tomorrow. Educate yourself. Make decisions based on what you believe is the best course of action for YOU.

Choose to create a quality life, balanced and fulfilled with *Winning Formulas for Health, Vitality, Longevity and Fat Loss.* This transformation begins with a thought and desire to adhere to improvements in your diet, thought patterns and other aspects of your lifestyle. Thought plus feeling equals emotion. Your beliefs and perceptions become your reality. Change your belief and you can transform your life.

George Bernard Shaw, Winner of the 1925 Nobel Prize in Literature quotes, "when you change the way you look at things, the things you look at change."

Anytime you want to change your life, you must change what you demand of yourself and raise your standards. Uproot old beliefs and replant new ones.

Find people and mentors who have a healthy relationship with food, lifestyle, exercise, admirable values and positive attitudes. Studies show that people do their best with a mentor. You may wish to start a *POWER OF 4* support group.

Surround yourself with like-minded individuals who make you feel good when you're with them. You are the sum of the five people you spend the most time with. Does this buddy, role model or expert enhance the quality of your life? Does he or she inspire and motivate you to be your best self?

Focus on becoming as healthy as possible – way down to the cellular level – because in the long run you can only look as good on the outside as you are healthy on the inside. Thinking this way, and making choices based on what will actually make you healthier today, tomorrow and for the rest of your life will change your way of eating, exercising, thinking, resting and breathing – permanently. The result will be life changing.

There will be those occasions when a setback is experienced. Instead of giving up and quitting, consider this to be part of the human experience. Make up your mind to get back on track immediately. Direct your attention and focus on what you did positively to achieve your goals that day.

As you turn the pages of this book, I will share with you my philosophy from years of experience on the topics of nutrition, lifestyle, exercise and supplementation. Provided herein are easy, reliable, ready-to-implement solutions – *Winning Formulas* – for a lifetime of *Health, Vitality, Longevity and Fat Loss.*

CHAPTER 2-1

THE POWER OF NUTRITION

READ INGREDIENT LABELS

"Let food be your medicine and medicine your food. Whosoever gives these things no consideration and is ignorant of them, how can he understand the diseases of man?"
~Hippocrates

If you cannot pronounce it and don't know what it is, don't put it in your mouth! That's right. What you don't know may hurt you.

As a rule, the most significant detail to pay attention to is the ingredient statement on a product, not the macronutrient breakdown (protein, carbohydrates and fats). Clever marketing and advertising distracts most individuals to bypass this important *Winning Formula* – read the list of ingredients. Marketers highlight what they want you to notice. Products labeled "organic, sugar-free, low-fat and cholesterol-free" can all be deceptive and misleading.

Allow me to enlighten you regarding a few of the ingredients you'll find listed in many of your every day beverage and food products.

ARTIFICIAL FOOD COLORING

How prevalent is artificial food coloring? Take a look in your pantry or medicine cabinet. Everything from cereals, sports drinks, lotions and shampoos, to over-the-counter and prescription medicines contain artificial food coloring. Kellogg has removed the dyes from Nutri-Grain cereal bars sold in the U.K., but not those sold in the U.S. There are nine artificial colors approved for use by the FDA!

In Dr. Ben Feingold's book, *Why Your Child Is Hyperactive,* he states, "that there is a definite link between hyperactivity and food coloring." An article published in *The Lancet* in September 2007 confirmed "a link between food dyes and ADHD."

Whenever you see a color followed by a number in the list of ingredients, this is an indication to avoid that product. These include red #3 and #40, yellow #5 and #6, blue #1 and #2 plus green #3. Ingredients such as yellow #6 have been linked to possible kidney and adrenal tumors. Yellow #6 has been banned in Sweden and Norway.

Yellow #5 is the most notable color agent because it causes the most immediate allergic reaction in those sensitive to salicylates, such as aspirin. You will find yellow #5 in Kraft Macaroni and Cheese, Eggo® Waffles, ice cream, cereals, candy, spaghetti, gelatin and puddings.

Red #40 is used in foods, drugs, pet food, cosmetics, soda and candy. It is a suspected carcinogen. There are four documented deaths related to red #40 coloring agent. Gatorade® Fruit Punch, strawberry Pop-Tarts®, Fruit Loops®, Nutri-Grain® Blueberry bars, Tylenol® Plus Cold Infant Drops, Flintstones™ vitamins and red M&Ms® contain red #40.

If you require food coloring for a specific recipe, you can find healthier alternatives such as extracts of turmeric, blueberry and beet at your health food store.

SODIUM NITRATE

Sodium nitrate is found in a variety of luncheon meats, ham, bacon, corned-beef, hot dogs and sausages. This chemical preservative gives meat its bright red color, prolongs shelf life and kills *Clostridium botulinum* spores (botulism). When consumed, this chemical preservative combines with your natural stomach chemicals forming nitrosamines. Nitrosamines are powerful carcinogens – causing cancer.

SOYBEAN OIL

Watch out for partially hydrogenated soybean oil. You'll find hydrogenated soybean oil in every product imaginable! The hydrogenation process alters the configuration of the fat molecule, creating trans fatty acids, which are detrimental to your health. They have been linked to heart disease. Trans fats interfere with normal fat metabolism. (Read about trans fats in Chapter 2-3.)

ARTIFICIAL SWEETENERS

The FDA refused to approve the artificial sweetener, NutraSweet™, for many years because it was known to induce brain cancer and seizures. It is now in over 7,000 foods!

Splenda® is our nations' number one selling artificial sweetener. It is marketed as a "healthy and natural" sweetener. Splenda, a man-made substance, is the brand name for sucralose which is a chlorinated sugar molecule. Splenda equals sugar plus three chlorine atoms. It was supposed to be an insecticide. Chlorine is a deadly poison. It was used in its gaseous form to kill people in World War I. Your DNA does not recognize the coding for assimilation or for usage and therefore, is not metabolized.

Splenda disrupts the central nervous system creating a feeling of comfort from eating sweet foods, which leads to addiction. The chlorine builds up in your system creating a toxic load.

It is proven that there is a connection between harmful, artificial sweeteners, synthetic food additives, preservatives and ADHD. Ritalin is an amphetamine which causes addiction and brain cell death. We are not a Ritalin deficient society! Other side effects of ADHD drugs include skin rash, nausea, insomnia, disrupted heart rhythm, aggression and psychosis. Avoiding synthetic food additives, preservatives and artificial sweeteners improve ADHD symptoms.

Splenda® side effects from animal testing include:

- Aborted pregnancy; decreased fetal body weights and placental weights
- Atrophy of lymph follicles in the spleen and thymus
- Decreased red blood cell count
- Diarrhea
- Enlarged liver and kidneys
- Extension of the pregnancy period
- Hyperplasia of the pelvis
- Reduced growth rate
- Shrunken thymus glands (up to forty percent shrinkage)

Aspartate, a neurotoxin, is a major component in the artificial sweetener, aspartame. Aspartame is a mixture of two amino acids, phenylalanine and aspartate, plus methanol (wood alcohol). Both of these amino acids are capable of converting to the neurotransmitters, dopamine and norepinephrine. Aspartame over-stimulates the brain neurons to the point of killing them. Need I go on?

If a pregnant woman drinks large quantities of diet soda, which is full of aspartame, her placenta may accumulate methyl alcohol, causing mental retardation in the fetus.

People consuming artificial sweeteners risk malnutrition because of the gastrointestinal problems and diarrhea associated with artificial sweeteners.

It's quite ironic that so many individuals drink soft drinks with aspartame, (i.e., NutraSweet®) when aspartate can produce the exact same dysfunction as glutamate, resulting in gross obesity.

Products with artificial sweeteners are denatured, altered, processed and full of man-made chemicals which damage your cells. Everything from soda and chewing gum to desserts and yogurt contain aspartame. Some vitamins and cough drops also contain aspartame. Always read the list of ingredients.

There are over ninety side effects from ingesting aspartame. Some of the side effects you may experience from aspartame include: water retention, increased appetite, weight gain and excessive stimulation of brain cells causing them to die.

Aspartame may cause rashes, neurological diseases, muscle pains, diabetes, headaches, dizziness, numbing of extremities, seizures, emotional disorders, hypertension, depression and birth defects. Aspartame poisoning mimics symptoms of MS.

Long-term consumption may predispose an individual to Parkinson's disease, Multiple Sclerosis or Alzheimer's disease.

Are you ready to give up your diet soda yet? Allow me to further enlighten you.

Artificial sweeteners added to soft drinks are linked with testicular damage. Just one diet soda can kill brain neurons within six to eight hours and regular consumption can cause brain damage and cancer.

Aspartame accounts for more than seventy-five percent of the total adverse reactions to food reported to the U.S. Federal Drug Administration. Hundreds of airline pilots have reported symptoms of memory loss and confusion, headaches, seizures, visual disturbances and gastrointestinal problems as a result of consuming artificial sweeteners.

A recent review published in the *European Journal of Clinical Nutrition* found aspartame to have a significant weakening impact on your brain, setting you up for problems ranging from mental and emotional disturbances to learning disabilities.

According to this May 2008 study, "aspartame appears to cause both direct and indirect changes in brain chemistry." The researchers found that among other negative side effects, "aspartame can disturb your brain's ability to metabolize amino acids and proteins." This revealed that aspartame damages the integrity of nucleic acids and interferes with the functioning of neurons. The research team concluded that "excessive aspartame ingestion might be involved in the pathogenesis of certain mental disorders as well as compromised learning and emotional functioning."

Are you willing to sacrifice your health, and your mental and emotional function to save calories? Save yourself the risk and switch to stevia, a natural sweetener. (See page 64.)

MONOSODIUM GLUTAMATE (MSG)

MSG is a food additive commonly used by the food industry to enhance the flavor of their product. MSG is a major culprit in chronic disease and has been linked to numerous health problems.

Glutamate in its free form is an excitotoxin. In animal studies, excitotoxins have been shown to cause neurotoxicity as well as weight gain.

MSG can induce migraines in adults as well as children. Food manufacturers are adding MSG to foods in ever growing amounts. MSG addicts people to the products that contain the additive. It is in everything from formula to vaccines to supplements.

MSG is allowed in food products for babies and children. "Hypoallergenic formulas tend to contain more MSG than traditional formulas," according to a 2002 Canadian study.

Supplements are another product that can expose individuals to MSG. A number of brands of fish oils, encased in gelatin capsules, various soy and whey protein powders and Flintstones™ vitamins contain MSG or aspartame.

Even though the word MSG is not on the ingredient listing – "buyer beware." This is no guarantee that the product or item is void of "excitotoxins." MSG may be hidden in one of the other ingredients.

These ingredients contain MSG:
<ul><li>Autolyzed vegetable protein</li><li>Autolyzed yeast extract</li><li>Bouillon</li><li>Calcium caseinate</li><li>Cornstarch</li><li>Gelatin</li><li>Hydrolyzed vegetable protein</li><li>Malted barley</li><li>Sodium caseinate</li><li>Soup base</li><li>Textured vegetable protein</li><li>Textured whey protein</li><li>Vegetable protein extract</li><li>Yeast extract</li></ul>

MSG has been linked with reduced fertility as well as obesity in several studies conducted in Germany.

Studies recommend "excluding MSG from your diet as it has the potential to damage the hypothalamic regulation of appetite. MSG may also trigger asthma."

A ten-week study conducted in Canada had families eliminate artificial colors, MSG and preservatives. More than half of the children in these families showed significant improvements in behavior, as well as improved sleeping, night waking and halitosis.

In the medical journal, *Archives of Disease in Childhood*, a study revealed the effects of artificial preservatives and food additives on the behavior of 400 children. The results demonstrated "a substantial effect" of these synthetics stimulating hyperactivity and behavioral problems.

HIGH-FRUCTOSE CORN SYRUP (HFCS)

Another deadly sugar substitute is high-fructose corn syrup (HFCS). HFCS is sugar produced by processing corn starch to yield glucose, and then processing the glucose to produce a high percentage of fructose. HFCS has much higher quantities of fructose than fruit, without the natural fiber that slows digestion and feeds the beneficial bacteria. With HFCS, only the harmful bacteria gets fed and gastric distress becomes inevitable with an end result of indigestion, acid reflux and irritable bowel syndrome.

HFCS has become increasingly popular because it is very inexpensive to produce. Due to the sweetness of corn, your appetite AND your weight increase!

Consuming high-fructose corn syrup not only exacerbates obesity, it increases inflammation and oxidative stress. HFCS predisposes a person to bone loss, anemia and heart problems. HFCS damages your organs, particularly the liver and pancreas.

HFCS radically spikes insulin and blood sugar while halting the biological production of anti-aging and muscle building hormones. Even worse, HFCS gives rise to deadly AGE (advanced glycation end), age accelerating molecules, causing you to overeat. AGE molecules are responsible for causing unsightly wrinkles and age-related blindness.

You'll find HFCS in a variety of processed foods such as salad dressings, crackers, soft drinks and various fruit drinks. Beware of high-fructose corn syrup in its disguised form. It may be on the ingredient label listed as glucose fructose syrup, fruit fructose, inulin and others.

Raw honey is a healthier choice for a sweetener, although not advisable for diabetics or those intolerant to carbohydrates.

A wonderful alternative to artificial sweeteners is an extract of the herb stevia. Stevia is a safe sweetener that will not disrupt your blood sugar levels and it has zero calories. Stevia is the ***Winning Formula*** sweetener for diabetics.

The short-term and long-term side effects from ingesting these toxic chemicals are not worth it. Always read the list of ingredients. Eliminate products containing:

- Artificial food colorings (Any color with a number after it)
- Artificial sweeteners: phenylalkaline, saccharine, aspartame and sucralose (all items ending in <u>ose</u>)
- BHA and BHT
- High-fructose corn syrup (HFCS)
- Monosodium glutamate (MSG)
- Sodium nitrate
- Soybean oil and all partially hydrogenated oils (trans fats)

Supermarket shelves are stocked primarily with processed, packaged foods. At least ninety percent of them contain some sort of refined sugar or carbohydrate. Foods that are refined and processed are taken out of their natural context destroying vitamins, minerals and important nutrients. First, reading labels, and knowing what to look for on them is crucial. If a product contains items such as partially hydrogenated oils, high fructose corn syrup, soy bean oil, aspartame, dextrose and enriched flour, don't buy it. Beware of any processed food because chemicals are always used. Shopping along the outer edges of the grocery store where fruits, vegetables and meats are usually located will make avoiding the packaged stuff a little easier.

CHAPTER 2-2

THE POWER OF NUTRITION

WATER AND HYDRATION

"What we give, we will receive and what we withhold will be withheld from us. The universe will always support our integrity."
~Marianne Williamson

Water is the primary energizer of all your bodily functions. Your body is composed of seventy-five percent water. Your brain tissue is approximately eighty-five percent water. Just a two percent reduction in water can create feelings of fatigue. A ten percent reduction in water causes significant health problems.

Water properly hydrates your spine and muscles, stimulates digestion, enhances optimal performance, encourages weight loss, transports nutrients, empowers your body's natural healing process, regulates body temperature, removes wastes and eliminates toxins. Water is a vital **Winning Formula** for health.

People suffering various health problems would definitely benefit from water with salt as a natural medication. However, not just any kind of salt will do. Unprocessed, Celtic sea salt is your best option. Celtic sea salt creates a healthy, alkaline environment instead of an unhealthy, acidic environment in your body.

Adding a pinch of sea salt to your drinking water encourages an increased absorption of water because it restores electrolyte balance. Celtic sea salt supports adrenal health.

Regular table salt is ninety-eight percent sodium chloride and two percent chemicals. Highly processed foods are loaded with sodium chloride. Consumption of table salt causes your body to retain fluids. This can result in kidney and gallstones, rheumatism, arthritis, gout and cellulite.

Celtic sea salt is a **Winning Formula** for those of you suffering from asthma because sea salt is a natural antihistamine, as well as a mucous breaker. Adding sea salt to your water and food fools your brain into thinking a great amount of salt has arrived in your body. It is then that your brain begins to relax the bronchioles.

The best sea salt is 100 percent unprocessed, Celtic sea salt (grey, beige or pink in color). The color indicates a high moisture level and trace mineral content. Quality Celtic sea salt will be void of heavy metal toxicity. Celtic sea salt is a good source of usable iodine as well, which helps boost the thyroid.

Adding the juice from lemon or lime to your water and/or food alkalizes your blood. The more alkaline you are the less cortisol you produce. Cortisol is a steroid hormone made in the adrenal glands. When you release high amounts of cortisol, your body switches over to producing primarily stress hormones rather than sex hormones.

Insufficient water intake causes dehydration which impacts your immune system negatively, lowers oxygen in your body and creates an acidic environment. These are prime conditions for cancer cell development.

Consume an adequate amount of water on a daily basis. The number of ounces required is different for each one of us. Traditionally, the recommendation is to drink eight glasses of water daily. This does not take into account the weight of the individual, activity level or environmental factors.

To calculate the number of ounces you need, take your bodyweight in pounds and multiply by 0.7. This formula will provide you with the number of ounces to drink daily.

Drinking water first thing in the morning assists in flushing your digestive tract.

Lack of water consumption may contribute to the formation of kidney stones by concentrating the calcium salts inside the kidneys. An increased risk of kidney stones is also associated with a high consumption of high-fructose corn syrup.

The color of your urine should be a very light colored yellow, similar to lemon juice. If it is a deep, dark yellow color, like that of apple juice, this is an indication that you are not drinking enough water. Note that vitamin B2, riboflavin, may produce bright, fluorescent-yellow colored urine.

Signs and attributes of dehydration:

- Allergies and asthma
- Arthritic pain and low back pain
- Constipation
- Dark colored urine with a strong odor
- Elevated cholesterol and high blood pressure
- Excessive weight
- Headaches
- Inability to concentration
- Increased acidic environment (prime for development of cancer cells)
- Insomnia
- Kidney stones
- Lower abdominal bloating
- Reduced motivation and performance

Drinking room temperature water versus ice-cold water has its advantages. Room temperature water improves your body's ability to absorb water far superiorly to ice-cold water because room temperature water enters your muscles faster.

You can make your own electrolyte replenishing drink with Celtic sea salt, a small amount of fresh, organic juice and distilled water.

Health problems including cancer of the colon, kidney, bladder and breast may be related to unintentional water deficiency. This creates a highly acidic and low oxygen environment. Cancer cells thrive in this type of environment. Water flushes toxins from your body before the toxins can execute their damage or be re-absorbed.

Drinking water is often available in plastic containers. Americans consume fifty micrograms of plastics daily! Gradually make the switch to glass bottled water versus a plastic bottle to avoid consumption of xenoestrogens and various chemicals.

Our food supply contains petrochemical residues from plastics, which have estrogen-like endocrine disrupting effects in animals and humans. These substances have been linked to hormone-sensitive cancers including endometrial, breast and prostate cancer. Furthermore, plastics inhibit your thyroid gland, increase estrogen and decrease testosterone.

Bisphenol-A (BPA) is a chemical used in the manufacture of common polycarbonate plastic products including baby bottles and water containers.

A report by the *Science Daily Journal* disclosed that the amount of bisphenol-A (BPA) that leaches from plastic bottles into the drinks they contain is dependent upon the temperature of the liquid. When plastic drinking bottles were exposed to boiling hot water, BPA was released fifty-five times more rapidly.

BPA has been shown to disrupt hormones, affect reproduction and brain development.

German researchers have found that "the longer a bottle of water has been sitting on a store shelf or in a household pantry, the higher the dose of antimony, a potentially toxic trace element, it contains." The concentration was even higher after the bottles were left at room temperature for six months or exposed to sunlight.

If you live in a warm climate you can only imagine the toxins that excrete into your water bottles while being stored in various warehouses during the summer season!

In April 2008 the National Toxicology Program (NTP) raised concerns that "exposure to BPA during pregnancy and childhood could impact the developing breast and prostate, accelerate puberty and affect behavior in American children." Days later the Canadian government decided to label BPA as "toxic."

Yale School of Medicine researchers report that low doses of the environmental contaminant bisphenol-A (BPA) used to make many plastics found in food storage containers can lead to learning disabilities in children and neurodegenerative diseases in adults.

Studies indicate that "nearly every American is exposed to BPA chemicals, and that infants and children are at the highest risk for toxicity caused from BPA exposure."

Exposure to BPA may be associated with increased risks of avoidable morbidity, including cardiovascular disease, diabetes, Parkinson's disease and abnormal levels of liver enzymes.

Studies show "canned foods are a predominant source of daily BPA exposure in our lives." Food and drink cans are lined with a BPA-containing plastic. Beverages appear to contain less BPA residues, while canned pasta and soups contain the highest levels.

The Environmental Working Group (EWG), a nonprofit organization, found that "the worst foods tested put pregnant women and formula-fed infants within an unacceptable margin of safety to levels that cause harmful effects in laboratory animals."

The Environmental Working Group (EWG) continues to call for federal agencies to fully assess the safety of children's BPA exposures from formula, baby bottles and other sources.

Winning Formulas to reduce your exposure to Bisphenol-A

- Discontinue purchasing canned foods and beverages
- Eliminate plastic wrap
- Never microwave food in plastic containers
- Store food and beverages in ceramic and glass containers
- Use glass dishes, water bottles and baby bottles

There are various companies who distribute their water in glass bottles. Choose glass over plastic bottles for water. You can refill the glass bottle with your filtered reverse osmosis water from home – and, add a pinch of Celtic sea salt, of course.

Water functions as a *Winning Formula* to:

- Carry oxygen and nutrients to cells
- Cushion organs and tissues
- Empower your body's natural healing process
- Flush out toxins through kidneys and liver
- Help maintain weight
- Hydrate your spine and muscles
- Lower cholesterol
- Lubricate joints and protect your spinal cord
- Promote digestion and helps prevent constipation
- Regulate body temperature
- Serve as the medium for all energy reactions in your body
- Transport minerals throughout cells of the body

CHAPTER 2-3

THE POWER OF NUTRITION

SMART FATS

"Whatever we focus on is bound to expand. Where we see the negative, we call forth more negative. And where we see the positive, we call forth more positive. Having loved and lost, I now love more passionately. Having won and lost, I now win more soberly. Having tasted the bitter, I now savor the sweet."
~ Marianne Williamson

Is your goal to lose body fat? You must eat fat in order to lose fat. Ironic as it may seem, including adequate amounts of smart fats in your diet encourages fat loss. Individuals whose diets are too low in fat tend to consume a diet high in sugar and vice versa.

Fat is required for optimal hormonal function. Our medical community, along with the majority of the American population, has become so misled about the relationship of dietary fat and normal physiology. Decreasing dietary fat intake too low will result in increased mortality from cardiovascular diseases.

The human brain is the fattest, most cholesterol-rich organ in your body. Cholesterol is good! Imagine that?

Cholesterol is a necessary part of every cell in your body and is essential in virtually all aspects of metabolism.

Cholesterol is manufactured in the liver. Cholesterol exists in every cell of your body as a fat-like substance. You do not have a cholesterol level in your blood. Cholesterol is insoluble in blood, and therefore has to be carried around the body inside a small sphere known as a lipoprotein.

Cholesterol is necessary for your brain, nervous system, hormones, digestion, liver function, heart muscle contraction, calcium metabolism, bone structure and skin. Cholesterol forms fifty percent of your nervous system and serves as the conductor of nerve impulses. Cholesterol is so important that your body produces four to seven times as much as you ingest and reduces its production to accommodate cholesterol intake from the food you eat. Low cholesterol levels result in a compromised immune system, depression and many more imbalances.

We have been brainwashed by the American Medical Association (AMA), the Food and Drug Administration (FDA), Big Pharma, the media and physicians that we're a statin-deficient society. We're told that elevated cholesterol levels lead to heart disease. Russell L. Smith, Ph.D., author of *The Cholesterol Conspiracy* states, "Both the public and clinical physicians have simultaneously been swamped by an ever-growing tidal wave of exaggerations, distortions and even fabrications of the facts."

Jane Heimlich began extensive research on this cholesterol issue in 1989. In her book, *What Your Doctor Won't Tell You*, she concludes, "there is no question that the cholesterol program benefits three powerful groups in our society to the tune of billions of dollars. These three are the food companies, the pharmaceutical industry and the medical profession."

Adverse effects of taking statin drugs include:

- Brain fog and dementia
- Cancer
- Depletion of CoQ10 enzyme
- Depression
- Heart failure
- Muscle and joint pain; muscular weakness
- Parkinson's
- Swelling of the face, lips, throat or tongue

Predisposing factors that contribute to elevated cholesterol levels may be from lack of exercise, consumption of too many starchy carbohydrates and hydrogenated fats, inflammation, leaky gut syndrome, obesity, endocrine and liver/biliary dysfunction or excessive stress in the form of physical, nutritional, chemical, electromagnetic and psychological.

Simple *Winning Formulas* to lower cholesterol levels naturally include eating more high-quality fats such as coconut oil, avocados, extra-virgin olive oil and supplementing with high-grade omega-3 fish oil.

A placebo-controlled study indicated that "supplementation with higher doses of fish oil may lower levels of plasma triglycerides naturally." (See Chapter 5-2 for more on fish oil.)

Reducing your intake of sugar and refined grains, which are omega-6 fatty acids, will result in decreased triglycerides. Consuming excess grains, refined carbohydrates, sugar and alcohol creates additional inflammation which increases cholesterol, especially triglycerides.

Cholesterol is a *Winning Formula* for:
• Fat and mineral absorption
• Forming the myelin sheath around all nerves
• Optimal functioning of serotonin receptors
• Optimal immune functioning
• Powerful antioxidant to control free-radical damage
• Precursor to sex hormones, vitamin D and bile production
• Production of all adrenal hormones

A great deal has been spoken and written concerning the evils of increased cholesterol; however, little has been reported concerning decreased cholesterol. Many studies reveal "a higher death rate in the elderly who have lowered cholesterol levels." Elderly females with cholesterol levels below 155mg/dL are associated with a 5.2 times higher death rate as compared to women with a cholesterol level of 272mg/dL. If your cholesterol level drops below 150mg/dL, it is possible you will suffer adverse health problems such as Alzheimer's disease, Parkinson's and cancer. Decreased cholesterol can be normal for a vegetarian or those with a genetic predisposition. Studies suggest that total cholesterol levels below 180 mg/dL increase the risk of suicidal behavior, hemorrhagic stroke, depression, free-radical pathology and cancer. (JAMA, Dec 1980).

Optimal ranges for cholesterol as stated by Dr. Harry Eidenier, Jr., Ph.D.	
Total cholesterol	180-220
Triglycerides	40-110
HDL	A minimum of 55
LDL	0-120 with 156 being an alert high

Stress, a highly-refined diet and a chaotic lifestyle, as well as hormonal profiles and liver congestion are all factors to consider when reviewing an individual's lipid panel. Though scientists still link total blood cholesterol with the risk for cardiovascular disease, Ancel Keys, Ph.D., professor emeritus at the University of Minnesota 1997 quotes, "there is no connection between fat intake and cholesterol – in fact, quite the reverse."

Establish a balance of omega-6 to omega-3 ratios by increasing your intake of smart omega-3 fats. An ideal omega-6 to omega-3 ratio is 2:1 to 1:1. The typical American diet is a ratio of 25:1 up to 50:1. Grain-fed beef, refined cereals and vegetable oils such as sunflower, safflower, corn and soybean are foods high in omega-6.

The human body is unable to synthesize omega-3. This essential nutrient must be consumed via food, supplementation or both.

Omega-3 food sources can be found in organic, cage-free eggs, wild salmon, mackerel, herring, sardines, pumpkin seeds, walnuts, fish oil supplements, hemp seed, ground flaxseed and krill oil.

Wild fish is a healthier option than farmed fish. Farmed fish have less beneficial fatty acid patterns compared to wild fish. Unfortunately, farmed fish are contaminated with antibiotics, higher levels of PCBs, dioxin and other toxic cancer-causing chemicals due to the feed used in fish farms.

Wild fish and shellfish are ideal sources of omega-3 fats (EPA and DHA). Fatty acid, alpha-linolenic acid (ALA), is another omega-3 fat found in walnuts, flaxseed, wheat germ, grass-fed beef and leafy greens.

Your body converts ALA to EPA → EPA converts to DHA. Unfortunately, this conversion is not efficient. Research shows that "less than fifteen percent of ALA converts to EPA and less than five percent converts to DHA under optimal conditions."

An intermediate fatty acid formed from linoleic acid in the pathway to arachidonic acid is gamma-linolenic acid (GLA).

GLA is a healthy omega-6, polyunsaturated fat found in several plant oils including borage oil, black currant oil and evening primrose. Supplementing with GLA may alter your body's production of hormone-like compounds called prostaglandins.

GLA supplementation may help ease breast pain tenderness, although it may take three menstrual cycles before you feel the effects and up to eight months for the supplement to reach its full effect.

Include raw, organic nuts or ground flax seed meal in your smoothies or oatmeal at breakfast. This is an easy technique to add extra quality, smart fats to your diet. Flax seed oil is highly overrated. Flax seed oil is alpha-linolenic acid (ALA), which is an inferior source of omega-3 due to the conversion factor. Ground, organic flax seeds have other health benefits as it is high in fiber.

A study of 115 post-menopausal women showed that a higher intake of lignans, antioxidant phytoestrogens found in flax and sesame, was associated with lower total body fat mass and improved glucose metabolism. Including ground flax in the diet is an essential part of any program for weight loss or management, and for improving control of blood sugar, especially for diabetes.

DHA requirements for the brain increase as you age. In a study of 939 older subjects "low omega-3 fatty acid levels were found to be associated with dementia." Unfortunately, two of the best food sources of omega-3 fatty acids, fish and shellfish, have been affected by environmental contamination. While mercury occurs naturally in the environment, it is the mercury released into the air from industrial pollution that is a health concern.

When mercury falls from the air and into the water it is converted to methylmercury, a form of mercury that can be harmful to an unborn baby or small child. This causes damage to the neurological system. Nearly all fish contain traces of methylmercury. The levels in tuna vary greatly among varieties. Light, canned tuna is not as high in mercury, while white albacore, canned tuna contains much higher levels, as do fatty tuna steaks. Wild salmon, cod, haddock, whitefish and catfish contain lower levels of mercury.

Symptoms and characteristics of essential fatty acid deficiency include hair loss, depression, asthma, weight gain, heart disease, learning disabilities, alcoholism, PMS and dry, cracked heels.

Let's look at vegetable oils. Included in this category are corn, soybean, sunflower, safflower, peanut, canola and cottonseed oil. Although these polyunsaturated fats are usually described as 'heart-healthy,' they are high in omega-6 fatty acids, highly processed and perishable. This means the fats become rancid quickly, contributing to oxidative stress and damaging free-radicals in your body. Canola oil is a genetically altered potential inflammation- and cancer- promoting omega-6 fatty acid.

Dr. Uffe Ravnskov, M.D., Ph.D., author of *The Cholesterol Myths,* cites a survey that showed "high consumption of polyunsaturated oils lead to premature aging."

Researchers at a San Francisco, CA hospital found that "babies admitted with conditions such as edema, anemia and blood cell disturbances were victims of commercial baby milk formulas containing skim milk and polyunsaturated oils."

When polyunsaturated oils are heated, as in food processing, they produce extremely reactive chemicals that can damage blood vessels, initiating atherosclerosis. The food industry prefers vegetable oils because they are less expensive.

The process of hydrogenation which transforms poly-unsaturated plant oils into solid fats is an extremely harmful process. These hydrogenated oils contain large amounts of toxic trans fats which have found their way into many processed foods.

Trans fats are poison. They interfere with the metabolic process of life. Eliminating all hydrogenated and trans fats, margarine and fried foods from your diet will reduce inflammation plus decrease free-radical production. Switch from margarine and butter substitutes to unsalted, organic butter and use Celtic sea salt.

Significant amounts of omega-6 intake create an imbalance that can interfere with the production of important prostaglandins. This may result in blood clot formation, increased inflammation, elevated blood pressure, digestive issues, depressed immune function, cancer, sterility, depression and weight gain.

Excess omega-6 fats have been shown to cause human prostate tumor cell cultures to multiply twice as quickly.

Olive oil, rich in monounsaturated fats, has been found to reduce the risk of atherosclerosis and increase HDL cholesterol. However, olive oil is very perishable. Olive oil is best eaten on salads and cold dishes, although not ideal for cooking.

Risk factors from eating trans fats/partially-hydrogenated fats

- Atherosclerosis
- Cancer
- Chronic high levels of cholesterol
- Decreased testosterone levels
- Diabetes
- Heart disease
- Increased inflammation and free radical production
- Liver damage
- Lower IQ
- Neurological and visual impairment of fetuses
- Obesity
- Osteoporosis
- Suppressed immune function

You've been convinced that saturated fats are unhealthy. Saturated fats are not the 'villain' fat. The key is to obtain your saturated fats from healthy food sources that aren't highly processed or contaminated with trans fats. Saturated fats protect against the harmful effects of trans fats!

According to the Weston A. Price Foundation, "saturated fats play important roles in body chemistry. They strengthen your immune system and are involved in inter-cellular communication, which means they protect us against cancer."

For calcium to be absorbed into your skeletal structure, fifty percent of the fats you consume should be saturated fats.

Dr. William Castelli, director of the Framingham Heart Study, observed "that the people who ate the most cholesterol, saturated fat and calories had lower serum cholesterol, weighed the least and were the most physically active."

A perfect example of a healthy, saturated fat is coconut oil. It is an extremely stable oil that contains a type of saturated fat called medium-chain triglycerides (MCT). MCTs are healthy for your immune system and intestinal health. They've been shown to support weight management. Because coconut oil is highly stable, it does not become damaged during high temperatures, making it the perfect oil for cooking.

Coconut oil, a healthy, functional fat, contains lauric acid which doesn't raise cholesterol. In addition, coconut oil has antibacterial, antiviral and antifungal properties. Coconut oil has the same qualities as that of breast milk.

A greater saturated fat intake is associated with less progression of coronary atherosclerosis, whereas excess carbohydrate intake is associated with a greater progression.

Research from several decades ago showed that eating the average American diet, with added coconut oil, demonstrated better measures of serum lipids than did the American Heart Association diet. It does not require the liver or gallbladder to emulsify it.

Coconut oil is very nourishing for the thyroid and the immune system. In addition, topical use of coconut oil is the perfect moisturizer for your skin. Coconut oil decreases cravings and stimulates your metabolism helping you to lose weight. Coconut oil has also shown antifungal benefits against *Candida albicans*, a type of yeast involved in vaginal yeast infections as well as thrush. Furthermore, coconut oil lowers cholesterol levels, improves insulin resistance and reduces your risk of heart disease. Research suggests that "coconut oil and fish oil are useful as therapies in acute and chronic inflammatory diseases."

Cod liver oil is at the top of the list for smart, healthy fats. Cod liver oil is rich in vitamins A and D. Cod liver oil has many of the same benefits of omega-3 fish oil, along with the myriad of benefits from vitamins A and D.

Use of cod liver oil in early life has been associated with a reduced risk of childhood-onset type 1 diabetes. A 2001 study in *Lancet* showed an eighty percent decrease in type 1 diabetes incidence in individuals who took 2,000 IU vitamin D daily during the first year of life.

Cod liver oil is highly effective for arthritis. Supplementation with cod liver oil, rich in omega-3 fatty acids, was found to reduce the required dosage of non-steroidal anti-inflammatory drugs (NSAIDs) for those individuals who use these drugs for inflammation and pain.

Dundee University researchers found that "supplementing with cod liver oil daily reduced the need for painkillers in people suffering with rheumatoid arthritis. A daily dose of ten grams of cod liver oil reduced the need for NSAIDs by thirty percent."

Reasons to include smart fats as a *Winning Formula for Health, Vitality, Longevity and Fat Loss*
• Correct gut dysfunction
• Decrease LDL cholesterol
• Hormonal balance
• Myelin sheath around nerves
• Natural anti-inflammatory
• Promote body fat loss (gives pancreas a break!)
• Protection from viruses and yeasts
• Protect liver from alcohol and other toxins such as Tylenol and other OTC drugs
• Reduce carbohydrate cravings
• Regulate insulin levels

CHAPTER 2-4

THE POWER OF NUTRITION

ELIMINATE ALLERGENS

"Everyone has a doctor in him or her; we just have to help it in its work. The natural healing force within each one of us is the greatest force in getting well. Our food should be our medicine. Our medicine should be our food."
~Hippocrates

Over seventy percent of the foods consumed in the Western diet didn't even exist ten thousand years ago. Many of us experience food intolerances or sensitivities without even realizing it. The top foods to which we encounter intolerances or sensitivities to include: sugar, wheat, gluten, dairy, casein, corn and processed soy.

Symptoms for both allergies and intolerances can be similar, such as involving the skin (e.g. hives, dandruff or eczema), respiratory system (e.g. asthma, bronchitis or congestion), nervous system (e.g. headaches or depression) or digestive tract (e.g. indigestion, diarrhea or bloating). However, a food allergy is an antibody reaction of your body's immune system to a food or food ingredient that your body perceives as foreign.

With a food allergy, your immune system may react quite violently to certain foods causing a great deal of distress to your body. Peanuts, nuts, fish and shellfish are common foods creating life-long allergies. Food allergies are a rather fast response (minutes) by the body's immune system to a perceived invader. Signs or symptoms are usually immediate, dramatic and visible such as coughing, sneezing, migraines, watering eyes, rashes, hives – or in severe cases anaphylactic shock which requires emergency intervention. Less than five percent of the U.S. population exhibits what is called a "true" food allergy.

Food intolerance is a slow onset reaction (hours, days or even weeks) to a certain food, food ingredient or additive that involves your immune system. It typically involves your digestive system. Food intolerance is an inability to properly digest certain foods.

When food sensitivities cannot be confirmed by standard allergy tests, it is called food intolerance. Thirty to ninety percent of individuals suffer from food intolerance.

Major symptoms of food intolerances consist of a long list of body ailments including: headache, lethargy, sleep disorders, hyperactivity, gastrointestinal problems, runny nose and sinus problems, mouth ulcers, urinary problems, weight fluctuation and obsessive (addictive) eating.

Food intolerances create additional stress on your body limiting the availability of serotonin.

Serotonin is a feel-good neurotransmitter that creates a positive mind-set. A serotonin deficiency has been associated with carbohydrate binging. Approximately ninety percent of serotonin is manufactured in your intestines.

When you continue to eat foods that your intestines are intolerant toward, your gut becomes inflamed. Oftentimes, those with addictive food sensitivities eat the very food that they are addicted to each and every day. In some people, their gastrointestinal tract is unable to produce appropriate enzymes for normal chemical breakdown. The food passes through unprocessed or lingers in the gut fermenting and producing excess gas. In some cases, protein fragments rupture the lining of the intestine allowing foreign particles into the bloodstream.

When you eat the intolerant foods you're addicted to, an adrenalin rush (the classic "fight or flight" response) is experienced. This is the 'hook' that keeps you coming back for more. Although you feel good for a short amount of time, the 'high' soon passes and you return to feeling drained and lethargic.

To avoid food intolerances, it is necessary to rotate your foods every day. Do not eat the same foods day after day. No food ought to be eaten more than every fourth day.

If the culprit food is one that you eat regularly, such as wheat or milk, and you omit it from your diet withdrawal symptoms may occur.

You may confirm any food sensitivity with a comprehensive blood test for IgG which measures antibody reactions. Food allergies are confirmed with IgE testing. Both of these tests are a convenient and easy way to diagnose food allergies and/or sensitivities.

The following conditions can be attributed to your diet:

- Arthritis
- Asthma
- ADHD
- Candida overgrowth
- Chronic sinus problems
- Dermatitis (skins problems such as hives, acne, rashes, rosacea)
- Depression
- Digestive disorders
- Fatigue
- Joint Pain
- Migraines and other headaches
- Overeating
- Obesity
- Repeat infections

GLUTEN

Gluten, a glue-like substance, is a protein portion of grains such as wheat, rye and barley. Gluten intolerance is common among people of Eastern Europe, Scandinavian, Scottish, Irish and English origin. Intolerance to gluten is associated with a family history of alcoholism, arthritis, Down's syndrome and mental disorders. Gluten intolerance is a major unrecognized risk factor for osteoporosis. Those with thyroid issues benefit immensely by eliminating wheat and gluten. Gluten intolerance is an autoimmune process, not a food allergy. Some common symptoms include fatigue, depression, increased inflammation, adult acne and weight gain.

More and more gluten-free products are showing up in the shopping aisles of your local supermarket due to a demand from gluten-sensitive individuals. The FDA now requires any source of wheat, the most common source of gluten, to be listed on the allergen statement located just below the list of ingredients. However, just because "wheat" is not listed on the allergen statement does not mean that it is "gluten-free" because gluten can also be found in products containing barley, rye and oats. Look for products with the "certified, gluten-free" seal.

DAIRY

"Milk does a body good?" Allow me to enlighten you. Health complaints associated with dairy intolerance include irritable bowel syndrome, allergies, acne and sinus problems. Side effects from dairy consumption can include everything from chronic ear infections in children to cancer and diabetes in adults.

Some people have an inability to tolerate milk because they lack the intestinal enzyme, lactase, which digests lactose (milk sugar), making them lactose intolerant. Most people stop producing lactase around the age of five.

Pasteurized milk strains your pancreas to produce enzymes. This places a tremendous amount of stress and tension on your body's digestive system.

According to the Weston A. Price Foundation: *"Pasteurization destroys enzymes, diminishes vitamin content, denatures fragile milk proteins, destroys vitamins C, B-12 and B-6, kills beneficial bacteria, promotes pathogens and is associated with allergies, increased tooth decay, colic in infants, growth problems in children, osteoporosis, arthritis, heart disease and cancer. Calves fed pasteurized milk do poorly and many die before maturity. Raw milk sours naturally, but pasteurized milk turns putrid; processors must remove slime and pus from pasteurized milk by a process of centrifugal clarification."*

Whole, raw milk from healthy animals can be a healthy alternative for some people. On the other hand, pasteurized milk may be full of assorted drugs and antibiotics, pesticides from treated grains, bacteria from infected animals and genetically altered growth hormones.

Dairy products tend to cause constipation. Homogenization of milk has been linked to heart disease. Those who drink milk may suffer from osteoporosis because dairy consumption creates an increased acidic environment in your body.

A Harvard study published in October 2001 looked at dairy product intake of over twenty thousand men. This study revealed that "men consuming a diet high in dairy had a thirty-two percent higher risk of developing prostate cancer."

Milk is not a great source of calcium that most people believe it is. In a Harvard nurses' study, 75,000 women were studied for twelve years and found that "those who consumed three or more glasses of milk per day, as compared with those who drank little or no milk, had significantly higher bone fracture rates."

Aside from the numerous health problems – such as allergies, osteoporosis and prostate cancer – associated with milk and dairy, there's an even more specific reason to eliminate milk from your diet. Researchers have found that "milk causes significant insulin secretion." In fact, milk and fermented milk products stimulate as much insulin secretion as whole wheat does.

People with many different healthy complaints notice a significant improvement when they avoid dairy. Green leafy vegetables are the best source of calcium on the planet!

Winning Formulas to prevent osteoporosis include:

- Adequate hydration/ water intake
- Avoid long periods without eating and low calorie diets
- Balanced hormones
- Consider vitamins D, K, B-12 and folic acid, iodine, omega-3 fatty acids and minerals, specifically magnesium and calcium
- Eliminate antibiotics, antacids, fluoride, diuretics and phosphorus intake (e.g. soda)
- Exercise (weight-bearing)
- Healthy nutrition: green leafy vegetables, prunes, raw milk, dried plums, kale, pineapple, tempeh, adequate protein
- Maintain a normal acid/alkaline pH (7.2)
- Minimize or avoid dairy products
- Avoid pharmaceutical drugs and "synthetic" supplements
- Reduce alcohol consumption
- Stop smoking
- Sunlight (20-30 minutes daily)

SUGAR

Have you ever been plagued by hard-to-diagnose health problems? You know something is wrong, but your doctor can't seem to figure out what's causing your health problem. You can't lose weight, no matter how hard you try, you feel depressed, can't sleep, feel sluggish, lack mental focus and have lost your libido. Well, it's not all in your head. The culprit? Sugar.

Sugar is more addictive than cocaine. Did you know that your immune system is suppressed for eight to twelve hours after consuming sugar? In 1821, each person consumed approximately ten pounds of sugar annually. Today, that number is an astounding 170 pounds of sugar per person annually.

Refined sugars cause and aggravate asthma, allergies, sinusitis, Candida overgrowth and migraine headaches. Eating sugar increases your appetite. Consuming sugar contributes to elevated blood pressure and increased cholesterol, particularly triglycerides, increasing your risk of heart disease. Sugar consumption amplifies pain and inflammation and also triggers mood disorders and depression. Excessive sugar consumption leads to obesity and type II diabetes. Excess sugar damages skin collagen and tendons. This promotes wrinkling of the skin – accelerating the aging process. Sugar depletes vitamins B and C from your body. Cracks in your lips and corners of your mouth are signs of vitamin B deficiency.

Regulation of your blood sugar is a major *Winning Formula* to avoid reactive hypoglycemia, obesity and type II diabetes. High blood sugar or high insulin levels lead to insulin resistance which is a pre-diabetic state. Tissues become less responsive to insulin. Insulin resistance is at an epidemic high in our society and continues to rise.

Insulin resistance occurs from excessive consumption of refined carbohydrates, sugar and alcohol, as well as altered hormone levels and high-stress lifestyles which leads to adrenal fatigue.

In these circumstances, insulin is released and blood glucose levels start to drop below the normal fasting levels. This causes the adrenals and liver to come to the rescue creating a condition known as reactive hypoglycemia. The liver releases stored glycogen.

Hypertension, a silent killer, is a rising health epidemic in our society. Those diagnosed with high blood pressure (hypertension) often have in conjunction, insulin resistance, heavy metal toxicity or both. The majority of these individuals have low blood levels of vitamin D. Hypertension at midlife is linked to significantly increased risk for Alzheimer's disease.

Reducing blood pressure does not happen overnight. Eliminating alcohol, refined sugars and refined carbohydrates are *Winning Formulas* for those with high blood pressure. Be patient, as it could take a few months before you see results.

According to a study by the American Society for Biochemistry and Molecular Biology, "sugary drinks like soda and some juices may increase your risk of Alzheimer's disease." The study also reveals, over the course of twenty-five weeks, the mice drinking the sugar-water had gained seventeen percent more weight than the regular-water mice. The mice drinking sugar-water had higher cholesterol levels. Every one of them developed insulin resistance. By the end of the study, the sugar-fed group had much worse memory and more than twice as many amyloid plaque deposits in their brains as the plain-water-fed mice. Amyloid plaque deposits are one of the hallmark characteristics of Alzheimer's disease.

Soda is the largest source of refined sugar in the American diet. The average American drinks fifty-five gallons of soft drinks annually! Soft drinks are a combination of phosphoric acid, sugar or aspartame, caffeine and tap water. Drinking just one soda daily increases your risk of diabetes and metabolic syndrome. Metabolic syndrome is characterized as high blood pressure, low HDL cholesterol, elevated triglycerides, obesity and insulin resistance. Hypertension, elevated cholesterol, obesity, type II diabetes and insulin resistance are all risk factors for Alzheimer's disease.

Diet soda is just as bad, if not worse than non-diet soda. One twelve ounce diet soda contains 180 milligrams of aspartame. Diet soda and diet foods alter your brain chemistry and metabolism, stimulating fat storage and weight gain.

One well-controlled, peer-reviewed seven year study found that "as little as twenty milligrams per day of aspartame can cause cancer in humans." Soda consumption leaches calcium from your bones; a major factor that contributes to osteoporosis. Some studies reveal that "cravings for sugar and alcohol intensify from drinking soda." Stimulating the brain of a child with these "pleasure-enhancing" chemicals in beverages will, in some cases, program their senses to look for and use stronger addictive substances such as hard drugs or large amounts of alcohol later in life.

Mary contacted me regarding her husband, Jeff. She was rather concerned about his ongoing complaints of joint pain and his excessive use of Ibuprofen. Jeff is a twenty-year-sober drug addict and alcoholic. Oftentimes, sugar replaces alcohol for recovering alcoholics. Jeff loved his soda. I suggested Jeff "try" a ten-day detox avoiding all sugar and soda. The first few days were extreme hell for Jeff. He felt miserable, feverish and experienced fatigue. The more toxic a person is when eliminating a toxic food, the stronger the healing process can be. The uncomfortable symptoms lasted four days. The fifth day Jeff was full of energy and free of toxic Ibuprofen. His pain diminished immensely! He has not touched a soda since, nor does he have the desire to do so after the positive results he attained following the principles of THE POWER OF 4.

Former alcoholics often replace alcoholic drinks with sweets and sodas without realizing that sugar plays havoc with their intestinal flora, fostering overgrowth of *Candida albicans* and other fungi. Under certain conditions, these pathogenic yeasts actually convert sugars in the gut to alcohol. There are well-documented cases of inebriation caused by sugar consumption and Candida overgrowth in persons who do not drink alcohol. The recovering alcoholic, in turning to sugar, is often supplying himself with alcohol throughout the day!

Fruit juices, another source of sugar-water, are calorically dense. Consider how many oranges you'd have to juice to make a glass of orange juice. The healthier option is the actual fruit. Fiber is provided in the fruit versus the juice, as well as an abundance of vitamins and minerals, especially organic fruit.

Gradually eliminate sugar and refined grains from your diet. This simple ***Winning Formula*** may provide astounding relief from body aches, pain and inflammation. Plus, you'll have more energy and lose weight.

Sugar intake is a strong risk factor that contributes to higher breast cancer rates, particularly in older women. Sugar feeds cancer. Refined carbohydrates and sugar consumption can aggravate your joints causing degeneration and create a highly acidic environment. Excess acids in your system do exactly what they sound like they do – they deteriorate and damage your cells.

Additionally, your body's survival mechanism will attempt to neutralize these acids. Consuming sugar, flours, grains and other refined carbohydrates creates an acidic overload in your bloodstream. The result is the beginning of degenerative arthritis, gout and a host of other health conditions.

Consider raw, unfiltered honey as a healthier alternative for a sweetener, although it should be used in moderation. Diabetics or those intolerant to carbohydrates should eliminate all sugars, including honey, and instead use stevia. Stevia is a natural plant leaf, high in antioxidants, with a delicious and refreshing taste. It's thirty times sweeter than processed sugar. Stevia was traditionally used by South Americans and Asians as a sweetener. Stevia helps maintain blood sugars, making it the ideal sweetener for diabetics. Stevia has zero calories. Stevia Plus™ green packets easily slip into your purse or briefcase. KAL and SunnyDew® are other quality brands of stevia. Even with stevia, you must read the list of ingredients!

Poor food choice is negatively associated with cravings, altered moods, alcoholism and/or depression. Consuming sugar encourages depression and mood disorders. Serotonin levels are affected by the selection of food you choose to eat. Rice and beans are one of the best *Winning Formula* food combinations to increase serotonin levels. In addition, exercise is a natural *Winning Formula* remedy for depression.

Proper food choice, supplementation and amino acid therapy are natural *Winning Formulas* to correcting brain chemistry, neurotransmitter deficiencies and amino acid imbalances for those suffering from depression or alcoholism.

If you experience any of the following, chances are probable that excess sugars, whether it's sugar from candies or sugar in the form of refined carbohydrates or alcohol, are to blame.

Symptoms of insulin resistance:
• Altered fasting serum glucose (optimum 80-95 mg/dL)
• Bloating – too many high-glycemic carbohydrates result in bloating and flatulence
• Brain fogginess – inability to focus
• Depression or mood swings – caused by ups and downs of blood sugar
• Elevated blood pressure
• Excess body fat, especially around the mid-section
• Fatigue and frequent sleepiness – some people are tired in the morning, some hit a low in the afternoon, and some are tired all day. You may also become sleepy after a meal.
• High triglycerides caused by over-production of insulin
• Low HDL cholesterol
• Wrinkles and prematurely aged skin

SOY

Soy contains phyto-estrogens, which are plant hormones. They are very similar to human hormones and can bind to estrogen receptors in your body. Menopausal women who have ovaries which no longer produce the estrogen they once did, may benefit from this hormonal boost, however for those with estrogen-sensitive tumors, over-stimulation of these receptor sites isn't wise.

Soy is present in virtually every processed food imaginable. Americans are eating soy in unprecedented quantities such as soymilk, soy burgers and soy ice cream. Meanwhile, some misinformed moms are still feeding their vulnerable babies soy infant formula, which exposes their child to the equivalent of five birth control pills worth of estrogen every day. For girls, this can cause premature development such as breast buds, pubic hair and even menstruation before age eight. In boys, this can retard sexual development and even cause learning disabilities. Soy is extremely toxic to infants. All infants should be fed breast milk the first year of life. The best substitute after breast milk is raw goat's milk. Soy formula should never be considered because soy-based formulas are high in phytoestrogens and other anti-nutrients. It is imperative that pregnant women avoid eating any soy because a high estrogenic environment in utero may increase the risk of breast cancer in the child.

Unfermented soy contains phytic acid, which has anti-nutritive properties and reduces assimilation of minerals such as calcium, magnesium, copper, iron and zinc. This inhibits absorption and creates disruption in the digestive system.

Most processed, unfermented soy products contain added flavorings, preservatives, sweeteners, emulsifiers and synthetic nutrients – a far cry from what you get after the traditional fermentation process that ancient cultures put their soy through before they would eat it.

Soy shrinks your brain. In a major ongoing study involving 3,734 elderly Japanese-American men, those who ate the most tofu during midlife had up to 2.4 times the risk of later developing Alzheimer's disease. The phytoestrogens from soy may increase your risk of dementia. However, tempeh, a fermented soy product made from the whole soy bean, has been associated with better memory. This could be related to the fact that it contains high levels of the vitamin folate, which is known to reduce dementia risk.

Soy inhibits your thyroid causing ↑ thyroid damage and disorders, especially in women. Soy phytoestrogens are potent anti-thyroid agents that cause hypothyroidism and may cause thyroid cancer. In infants, consumption of soy formula has been linked to autoimmune thyroid disease.

Although manufacturers of soy products have been allowed to label them "heart healthy," consumption of processed, unfermented soy foods like soy milk, soy meat, soy ice cream or soy energy bars does not come without side effects.

Consumption of refined soy products have been linked to:
<ul><li>Allergies</li><li>ADD (soy-based infant formulas contain eighty times more manganese than breast milk)</li><li>Cancer (breast, ovarian, prostate, uterine, thyroid)</li><li>Cognitive decline (shrinking of the brain faster)</li><li>Digestive problems and food allergies/intolerances</li><li>Increased toxic load (high amounts of pesticides from spraying and increased amounts of aluminum during processing)</li><li>Promoting kidney stones</li><li>Reduced assimilation of calcium, magnesium, copper, iron and zinc</li><li>Reproductive disorders</li><li>Thyroid dysfunction (due to high levels of goitragens)</li></ul>

Traditionally, in Asian cultures, soy was fermented before it was eaten. This not only makes the beans more digestible, it increases the nutritive properties while decreasing the presence of phytates. Meanwhile, these cultures ate soy in much smaller quantities (about two ounces a day) than the amount Americans eat.

If you drink a glass of soymilk, you are already drinking more soy than traditional cultures ate in a day. If you add to that a soy burger and some soy ice cream, you are eating an extreme amount of soy, the likes of which has never been consumed in history. Drinking only two glasses of soy milk for one month has enough phyto-estrogens to alter a woman's menstrual cycle.

Unlike in Asia where people eat small amounts of whole soybean products, Western food processors separate the soybean into two golden commodities – protein and oil. There's nothing safe or natural about this.

The high-tech processing methods of today fail to remove the anti-nutrients and toxins that are naturally present in soybeans. The high temperatures, high pressure, petroleum solvents, as well as alkali and acid baths cause toxic and carcinogenic residues to remain intact.

Daniel Sheehan, Ph.D., Director of the Estrogen Knowledge Base Program at the FDA's National Center for Toxicological Research says, "Isoflavones should be consumed cautiously."

The key to avoiding such health risks regarding soy is to stick with unprocessed, fermented varieties only.

A study in the June 2004 issue of *Carcinogenesis* found that "processed soy products and supplements may actually stimulate the growth of pre-existing, estrogen-dependent breast tumors, compared with whole soy foods." Soy foods contain high levels of aluminum which is toxic to your nervous system and your kidneys. Soy protein isolate contains aluminum, nitrates and MSG.

Partially, purified isoflavone-containing products may not have the same health benefits as whole soy foods. The researchers suggest that "it may be wise to avoid processed soy products and supplements that contain isoflavones," which is how most Americans consume soy. Instead, they said to choose minimally processed 'whole' soy foods.

While moderate consumption of traditional non-GMO soy is healthy for some, soy milk, soy sausage and soy ice cream are far from what nature intended and not desirable. If you're looking for a healthy approach to eat and enjoy soy, most experts agree that the following are beneficial, healthy soy options in moderation:

- Edamame
- Miso (fermented soybean paste)
- Natto (fermented soybeans)
- Naturally fermented soy sauce
- Tempeh (fermented soybean cake)

***Winning Formula* foods to include in your diet for
*Health, Vitality, Longevity and Fat Loss:***

All non-starchy vegetables

Apple cider vinegar

Avocado

Butter (organic, unsalted)

Celtic sea salt, spices and herbs

Coconut oil and coconut milk

Extra virgin olive oil, sesame and walnut oil

Fish: flounder, catfish, perch, herring, anchovies, mahi,
sardines, whitefish, haddock, cod, pollock and wild
salmon

Fruits including berries, lemons, limes, tomatoes, avocado

Goat milk

Grains (unprocessed): rice, brown rice, quinoa, millet,
buckwheat

Green drinks

Green tea, Yerba Mate Royale tea and other herbal teas

Herbs and spices

Legumes, lentils, beans (black, kidney, pinto, navy)

Non-fluorinated/chlorinated water

Non-GMO fermented soy

Nut butters

Nuts and seeds (raw)

Organic, wild cuts of meat such as buffalo and elk

Organic, free-range eggs

Organic, free-range poultry

Organic, grass-fed beef

Raw honey

Raw, organic, unpasteurized, non-homogenized milk from grass-red cows

Sweet potatoes and yams

Sweeteners: Stevia Plus or KAL stevia

Unsweetened nut milks (almond, hemp)

Various greens including romaine lettuce, spinach, collard greens, kale, dandelion, mustard greens

Eliminate the following items:

Alcoholic beverages (red wine okay, in moderation)

All refined, processed foods

All spray oils in a can

Artificial colorings

Aspartame, Sweet 'N Low, Equal, Splenda™

Bacon, luncheon, deli, hot dogs and processed meats

Bagels

Candies

Oils: vegetables, canola, sunflower, safflower, corn

Chewing gum

Cookies

Crackers, chips, pretzels

Enriched anything

Flavored coffee creams

Fluoride

Fried foods

Gluten products

Heavy metals (flu shots, deodorant containing aluminum)

High-fructose corn syrup

Instant products

Juice drinks and fruit juices

Low-fat and non-fat ice cream and/or yogurt

Mayonnaise

Microwave popcorn

Mints

Monosodium glutamate (MSG) products

Muffins

Non-fat and sugar-free products

NSAIDs and OTC medications

Oatmeal packets and processed cereals

Partially hydrogenated anything

Powdered soups

Rice cakes

Sleeping pills

Soda (diet included)

Sodium nitrates, sulfites and chemical preservatives

Soy (processed, unfermented, GMO)

Soybean oil

Soy sauce

Sugar

Sweetened yogurts (Dannon, Yoplait)

Tap water

Wheat and anything that says wheat

White bread

White flour

One of the most important *Winning Formulas* is to read the list of ingredients in a product.

CHAPTER 2-5

THE POWER OF NUTRITION

FOCUS ON QUALITY

"Consciousness is the ability to release the old and embrace the new with the awareness that all things end at the appropriate time and that all things begin at the appropriate time. Therefore, becoming conscious means living fully in the present moment, knowing that no situation or person will be exactly the same tomorrow."
~Caroline Myss

Focus on quality by choosing to eat organic foods. Organic foods are approximately forty times more nutritious than commercially farmed foods.

Forty-five plus years ago all of our foods were organic. An organic food is one that is grown without the use of pesticides, herbicides, fungicides, synthetic fertilizers, sewage sludge, genetically modified organisms or ionizing radiation. Organic meat, poultry, eggs and dairy products are produced from animals that are not fed antibiotics or synthetic growth hormones.

In October 2002, the Organic Trade Association (OTA) attracted attention with their findings from a breakthrough European Union study. This study found that "organic foods have a higher nutritional value when compared to non-organic foods."

Organic fruits and vegetables have up to forty percent more antioxidants than non-organically grown produce. Organic foods can reduce dietary pesticide ingestion by ninety-seven percent! Pesticides are linked to interference with sex hormones. Doctors that have been successful in using nutrition to treat cancer insist upon organic foods for their patients because of the higher quality nutrient content.

Remember this important *Winning Formula*: always read the list of ingredients. If it doesn't say the word "organic" in front of each and every word, "Buyer Beware." Just because something is organic does not make it a health food. An organic cookie loaded with sugar may have fewer pesticides, but it does not qualify as a healthy option.

The Environmental Working Group (EWG) is a nonprofit organization that examines pesticide levels in commercially grown produce. The EWG shopper's guide reveals which fruits and vegetables are lowest and highest in pesticide residues so you'll know which ones you should always buy as organic. (See Resources.)

According to the Environmental Working Group's most recent list, the following fruits and vegetables are most likely to be contaminated with pesticides:

- Apples
- Bell peppers
- Celery
- Cherries
- Grapes
- Lettuce
- Nectarines
- Peaches
- Pears
- Potatoes
- Spinach
- Strawberries

Washing fruits and veggies is a must-do every time you bring them home. Why? An overload of pesticides in air, food or water may set the stage for Parkinson's disease and possibly Alzheimer's disease decades down the road. Chemicals in pesticides can damage the energy-producing part of brain cells. There's also a pesticide and arthritis link.

Some fruits and vegetables scored lower in pesticides on the Environmental Working Group's scale. These include:

- Asparagus
- Avocado
- Bananas
- Broccoli
- Cabbage
- Corn (frozen)
- Eggplant
- Kiwi
- Mango
- Onions
- Pineapple
- Sweet peas (frozen)
- Watermelon

Organic fruit labels will have five digits beginning with the number nine. It is especially important to choose free-range and organic over non-organic when it comes to meats, eggs and dairy products. These foods have a higher fat content and toxins are stored in the fat. When your fat cells are full of toxins, your body produces more fat. Organic foods have a higher nutrient value required to detoxify your body.

Non-organic meats and dairy not only have chemicals from the environment, they also have chemicals that are intentionally given to the animals by the farmers. Half of all antibiotics sold in the United States are purchased by farmers. The FDA has given farmers permission to use bovine growth hormone (BGH) without disclosing this to consumers! Not only is BGH a detriment to the animals' health, BGH has an effect on your health as well.

Most of the animal foods found in supermarkets come from factory farms where the animals are fed processed soy, grains, concentrates made from animal remains, cement dust, plastic chips, plus other surprising ingredients. These animals are loaded with synthetic hormones and/or antibiotics. They're raised under stressful, inhumane conditions that affect the health of the animal as well as the health of the one who eats it. According to the USDA, "stress increases the animals' susceptibility to disease and reduces meat quality."

If your budget does not allow you to purchase organics meats and poultry, it is best to reduce your consumption of non-organic sources of animal protein.

Organic cattle are those that feed in an organic pasture primarily on grass, hay and legumes free from chemicals, pesticides and fertilizers. These animals are not fed anything containing genetically modified crops, growth hormone, plastic pellets, urea, manure or animal by-products.

Organic, grass-fed beef contains sixty-percent more omega-3s, 200 percent more vitamin E and two to three times as many conjugated linoleic acids (CLA), which protects you against heart disease, cancer and diabetes.

Organic, grass-fed beef and other organic products can be found at Trader Joe's, Jimbo's and Whole Foods. If these stores are not available in your area, you can purchase from an organic farm or an organic farmer's market. Otherwise, ordering online is an option. (See Resources.)

Consuming an organic diet before a child is conceived, during fetal growth and throughout adolescence will ensure a normal endocrine system, blood sugars, lipids and a healthy functioning immune system; eliminate toxic exposure to 180+ pesticides which are known to disrupt the development/functioning of the hormone system and establish a quality taste-based preference that is nutrient dense. Parental exposure to pesticides doubles the risk of childhood brain cancer. Organic farming produces nutrient-dense foods high in phytochemicals that contribute to weight management and disease prevention by providing a sense of fullness (satiety) which reduces excessive calorie consumption; decreases free radical damage to the cellular structure which in turn ↓ inflammatory diseases, risk of diabetes and cancer, plus slows and reverses neurological aspects of the aging process thereby increasing cognitive function and better memory.

You replace an average of 2,000,000 red blood cells every second. Your body's cells are constantly regenerating themselves. The substance they use to rebuild comes directly from the food you eat.

Focus on quality with this *Winning Formula*: start your day with a quality breakfast. Include an organic protein source. The first forty grams of protein you eat daily supports your immune system. Protein initiates thermogenesis (energy production through heat/fat burning) in your body.

A minimum requirement of one-half gram of protein per pound of body weight is sufficient for most adults. If you're active, an athlete or suffering from illness, your daily protein requirements increase – one gram of protein per pound of body weight for females; up to two grams of protein per pound of body weight for males.

Protein intake is a fundamental *Winning Formula for Health, Vitality, Longevity and Fat Loss.* Protein is required for every cell in your body. Your nails, hair and muscles are comprised of protein. You need protein to function optimally. It increases your metabolism. Protein will help you feel full longer. Proteins are rich in amino acids which help balance brain chemistry. Protein is required to build your body versus break it down. Protein is a necessary macronutrient for your ability to focus and concentrate.

Quality protein sources include: organic, free-range poultry and eggs, grass-fed beef and bison, whey protein isolate and wild fish.

Your body requires protein to prolong life. Your kidneys, brain, heart and every other vital organ all require protein. When there is insufficient protein available, your body will rob protein from other areas such as joint surfaces.

A study from the University of Massachusetts Medical School conveyed that "people who skipped breakfast regularly were 450 percent more likely to be obese than individuals who ate breakfast."

A study was done on lean, healthy women who maintained their normal exercise, activity and diet throughout the study. This study revealed that "when they skipped breakfast their cholesterol levels were affected. There was a decrease in HDL, an increase in total cholesterol and insulin levels were elevated."

If you exercise first thing in the morning without eating, you create an environment for increased body fat. (Muscle loss diet: Jog first thing in the morning on an empty stomach.) Your body requires adequate fuel. This is supplied from food.

Skipping breakfast affects your blood glucose levels. When blood glucose levels are low (for example, from skipping breakfast), or when the body has impaired use of glucose (as in diabetes), willpower is impaired.

Numerous studies confirm that "low blood glucose levels and poor glucose use are associated with lack of self-control as well as emotional and behavioral problems." In order to stabilize blood glucose levels, it is important for you to maintain a balance between two hormones, glucagon and insulin, which are produced by the pancreas and released by the pancreas every time you eat. Protein in the diet induces the production of some insulin and more glucagon whereas carbohydrates in the diet induce the production of lots of insulin and no glucagon. Insulin promotes fat storage. Glucagon burns fat.

Your energy levels, moods and how you feel throughout your day are indications of how you take care of yourself. The first thing you eat each day influences your neurotransmitters. This is reflected in how you'll feel and think the remainder of your day.

A quick and easy breakfast option could be a handful of raw, organic nuts or seeds and a protein smoothie (unsweetened almond or goat milk, berries and a hydrolyzed whey protein powder). A high-quality whey protein isolate will be free of lactose, making it the ultimate choice for a protein powder. Whey protein isolate is easy on your digestive system versus casein protein. Whey protein isolates contain protein concentrations of ninety percent or higher. During the processing of whey protein isolate, there is a significant removal of fat and lactose. As a result, individuals who are lactose intolerant find whey protein easier to digest.

Whey is a popular dietary protein supplement believed to provide antimicrobial activity, immune modulation, improved muscle strength and body composition, and prevention of cardiovascular disease and osteoporosis.

Extended periods without food causes hypoglycemia, adrenal fatigue and elevated insulin levels. This equals an increased body fat. Your muscles store glycogen, which is your stored fuel source – your brain does not.

The root of much depression, anxiety and other mental illness amongst women is not eating enough food to run their brain chemistry. Brain chemistry is disrupted, altering neurotransmitters such as serotonin and dopamine. Low calorie diets of less than 1800 calories per day deplete brain chemistry, increase body fat and cause metabolically active muscle tissue to atrophy.

Regardless of the time of day, eating approximately one hour before exercise ensures that glycogen (your muscles' stored fuel source) is available for performance. Your mental and physical energy depend upon how well you fueled yourself prior to your exercise session.

Due to the fast-paced, on-the-go schedules many of us live, we eat on the run, in our cars or while watching television. Opt to dine in a relaxed environment with a calm state of mind. Be conscious, mindful and present while eating. Your dining experience will be more enjoyable. You'll actually taste your food. As a consequence, you'll consume less food because you are aware of when you're truly satisfied. Try this simple exercise – eat with your eyes blindfolded or with your eyes closed. You will be amazed at the amount of food left on your plate because the visual element is eliminated, and your brain communicates to your stomach that it is satisfied. Get rid of the television, computer and other distractions that will trigger you to eat mindlessly.

For optimal digestion of food, it is healthier to eat your meals in a pleasant, peaceful environment versus a chaotic, stressful one. This means turning off the television and your cell phone. Avoid reading stressful news, listening to chaotic music or engaging in a stressful conversation while eating.

Drink approximately twelve ounces of room temperature water fifteen minutes before your meal. During your meal, drink only enough water to wash your food down. Drinking more than that during your meal dilutes hydrochloric acid concentrations in your stomach and weakens digestion. (See Chapter 5-1 for more on digestion and hydrochloric acid – HCl.)

Chew your food thoroughly (i.e.: approximately twenty chews for a piece of meat). Digestion begins in your mouth.

Set your utensil down after three or four bites of food. Breathe. Breathe again. Slow down and enjoy your food. If your food isn't thoroughly chewed nutrients are not absorbed. In addition, this causes your body to add fat because the nutrients are not broken down properly, inhibiting absorption. This causes your body to think you're depriving it, creating a sense of perceived famine. Digestion and assimilation of the food you eat improves tremendously when chewed thoroughly.

If you tend to experience any of the following within one hour of completing your meal, these are indications that the foods you consumed are not the appropriate choices for you:

- You develop a sweet craving
- You feel depressed, hyper, nervous, angry or irritable
- You still feel hungry, even though you are physically full
- Your energy level drops

Any of the above symptoms could also be associated to an improper combination of protein, fat and carbohydrates eaten at your last meal, as well as insulin resistance. (Read Chapter 2-4.)

There are various health benefits to a vegetarian diet such as fewer chemicals ingested and less complications with digestion. However, there are disadvantages of a vegetarian diet. The main disadvantage is that vegetarian diets lack in certain nutrients. Vegetarians are more likely to experience low iron levels, resulting in anemia. Red meat is the number one food source for iron. According to the Weston A. Price Foundation, a vegetarian diet is far from ideal mostly because it lacks animal fats. Scientific evidence shows that humans need animal foods, particularly animal fats, for optimum health.

Vegetarians are usually deficient in vitamin B-12 which can cause depression, fatigue and poor concentration. Elder individuals with lower than average B-12 levels were over six times more likely to experience brain shrinkage.

Vegetarian diets have been associated with reduced estrogen levels in females causing menstrual irregularities. Vegetarian diets are linked to decreased immune function leading to chronic health problems and eventually a damaged metabolism.

A Scandinavian study with 2,041 participants reported that people who ate little meat had the most symptoms of depression, tiredness and headaches (Larsson et al, 2002).

More specific personality characteristics have also been observed among vegetarians. These include feelings of inadequacy, fear and interpersonal distrust (Lindeman et al., 2000).

Potential nutrient deficits created from a vegetarian diet:

- B-12 and folic acid
- Calcium
- Creatine
- Inferior mineral status
- Low iron, iodine and zinc
- Lower amino acids values, especially taurine
- Omega-3 fatty acids
- Riboflavin (vitamin B2)
- Vitamin D

According to Olympic strength coach, Charles Poliquin, "in order for a vegetarian to decrease body fat they must supplement with carnitine."

Dr. Eric Serrano, M.D. states, "It is imperative all vegetarians supplement with a high-quality multi-vitamin and omega-3 fish oil."

While research and experts continue to battle it out whether vegetarianism is healthy or harmful, take comfort in knowing that we all have different needs. You must eat a diet that feels right for you and is ideal for you individually.

CHAPTER 2-6

WINNING FORMULAS FOR NUTRITION

"Knowing is not enough: we must apply. Willing is not enough: we must do."
~Goethe

Select two **Winning Formulas for Nutrition** from the list below or create your own. Write your two **Winning Formulas** down on a piece of paper or sticky post-it note where they will be visible to you. Make copies. Keep your **Winning Formulas** in several locations where you will see them.

- Add a pinch of Celtic sea salt to water.
- Allow a cheat meal every week.
- Are you eating a mixture of fresh, organic, steamed or raw vegetables daily? Fresh fruit? Fiber from vegetables and fruits help support bowel regularity and create an alkaline environment.
- Avoid foods with additives and chemicals.
- Avoid iron-deficiency anemia – include iron-rich foods and supplement with high-quality fish oil and multi-vitamin.
- Buy a juicer. Toss fruits and vegetables into the juicer.

- Choose a piece of fruit over fruit juices loaded with sugar.
- Choose fresh foods versus frozen or canned. The longer the shelf life, the more harmful it is.
- Choose olive oil and lemon or apple cider vinegar as salad dressing versus bottled dressings.
- Consume adequate amount of water for my body weight.
- Consume at least 20 grams (female) or 40 grams (male) of protein for breakfast.
- Consume grass-fed beef or cage-free, organic poultry and eggs.
- Consume more wild meats such as elk and buffalo.
- Cook foods in coconut oil.
- Cut down on the number of hormones and chemically altered foods.
- Cut out one type of unhealthy food every week.
- Discard all soda pop and unhealthy treats from your household.
- Do not eat two hours before bedtime.
- Don't overeat. Be mindful and stop when you're eighty percent full.
- Drink a bottle of spring water before lunch and another bottle of water before you leave work or school every day.
- Drink more green tea.
- Drink water from glass bottles versus plastic.

- Eat a quality breakfast of protein, fat and carbohydrates to fuel your brain, sustain your blood-glucose levels and optimize your metabolism.
- Eat five to six small meals daily, eating every three to four hours.
- Eat or snack every three to four hours.
- Eat when hungry.
- Eat within thirty minutes of waking.
- Eliminate "white" foods.
- Eliminate all artificial sweeteners.
- Eliminate refined carbohydrates.
- Eliminate sugar.
- Eliminate enriched wheat.
- Enjoy quality mealtime.
- Get the processed, chemically-laden foods and drug-like foods out of your house.
- Have a salad every day.
- Have your thyroid and adrenals tested by a qualified practitioner.
- Hold healthy-dish potluck celebrations.
- Identify your food intolerances, food allergies or food triggers.

- If diabetic or carbohydrate-intolerant, follow a diet that is low in carbohydrates and eliminate all refined carbohydrate food sources.

- If it does not run around in the field, swim, fly, or is not green – do not eat it.

- If vegetarian, consider supplementing with B-12, a high-quality multi vitamin and fish oil.

- Include more calcium-rich foods such as spinach and collards greens. Eliminate diary products.

- Include fiber-rich foods at your meals.

- Include more smart fats at each meal.

- Include more *Winning Formula* foods. (See pages 71-72.)

- Include organic protein sources at every meal.

- Increase serotonin naturally with a light, unrefined, carbohydrate-rich snack.

- Juice first thing in the morning instead of coffee.

- Keep a food journal for two weeks to pinpoint areas that need improvement.

- Make a list of your healthiest friends and schedule a lunch or dinner with them weekly.

- Pack your own lunch.

- Plan your weekly meals.

- Practice mindfulness and adhere to proper portion sizes – no super sizing.

- Practice portion control.

- Prepare cut up fruits and vegetables for healthy snacks.

- Read ingredient labels on all packaged products.

- Reduce your caffeine intake if you suffer from breast pain, swelling or lumpiness. Supplement with borage oil or evening primrose oil.

- Remove toxic, unhealthy fats from your diet.

- Remove trigger foods from your home.

- Replace margarine with organic, unsalted butter.

- Schedule an appointment with a naturopathic practitioner to test for food allergies.

- Set your fork down throughout your meal. Breathe.

- Shop for organic foods.

- Shop the perimeter aisles of your supermarket.

- Steam vegetables versus microwaving.

- Stock up on healthy snacks.

- Stop eating before you're full.

- Surround yourself with people who support your healthy goals.

- Try one new organic fruit or vegetable every week.

- Use stevia as your sweetener.

- When dining out, eat at a restaurant that serves healthy fare.

CHAPTER 3-1

THE POWER OF LIFESTYLE

SLEEP

"Sleep is a natural restorative, an antidote to the damage done to our bodies during the course of the day. It allows the body to replenish its immune system, eliminate free radicals and ward off heart disease and mood imbalances."
~Herbert Ross, D.C.

What if I told you that you could prevent your waistline from expanding, increase your memory, enhance your immune function, and reduce your risk of cancer?

Consider this – Do you get at least eight hours of restful sleep each night? Are your lights off at 10:00 p.m. (moon)? Do you get up no earlier than 6:00 a.m. (sun)?

According to the NIH (National Institute of Health), "physical repair to your body happens between the hours of 10:00 p.m. and 2:00 a.m. when you are asleep. Your mind (spiritual/emotional) repairs and regenerates between 2:00 a.m. and 6:00 a.m."

We seldom think of sleep as a *Winning Formula for Health, Vitality, Longevity and Fat Loss.*

Sleep stimulates and resets your hormones. Quality of sleep affects your immune system, memory and moods.

Sleep deprivation disturbs glucose metabolism, lipid profiles, androgen production and blood pressure. Sleep deprived individuals may develop dementia or Parkinson's disease.

Sleep disorders are often the result of poor diet, electromagnetic and emotional stress, hormonal imbalances, low serotonin levels, toxic overload and disrupted circadian rhythms due to jet lag and night shift work or 24-hour shift work, such as fire fighters.

People who sleep four hours or less per night are seventy percent more likely to be overweight and experience increased appetites. Sleeping less than four hours per night for just seven days accelerates the aging process.

Lost shuteye impacts your brain. You lose one IQ point for every lost hour of sleep you didn't get the night before. Sleep enables you to cope with and perceive stress in a healthy manner.

Your hormonal system is synchronized with the rising and setting of the sun. In the morning, the sun stimulates the production of cortisol, an awakening hormone. The natural release of the awakening hormone, cortisol, is released around 6:00 a.m. Your repair and regeneration hormones, melatonin and DHEA, elevate and release between the hours of 6:00 p.m. to 7:00 p.m. Cortisol levels in the body should be highest in the morning and taper off into the afternoon and evening.

Because of altered nutrition and lifestyle habits, this is reversed. This natural cycle can be disrupted by exposure to stimulants after 2:00 p.m., stressful events after hours, artificial lighting, computers and television. Oftentimes, this is the reason most people have a hard time falling asleep and staying asleep.

Fluctuations in testosterone during male menopause, known as andropause, may affect restful, quality sleep. (See Chapter 3-4 for more on hormones.) Additionally, wavering progesterone levels in peri-menopausal women may influence restful, quality sleep. If you have an adrenal issue and your cortisol levels are constantly elevated, quality sleep is never going to happen.

Sleep apnea affects one from experiencing quality sleep. Sleep apnea can create serious tension in a relationship due to the sleep loss suffered by the person who doesn't have sleep apnea.

Sleep apnea causes an individual to actually stop breathing which creates a tremendous amount of stress on their cardiovascular system. Sleep apnea happens when a blockage develops in the upper airway, preventing normal airflow. Sleep apnea could also be caused by a defect in the central nervous system, which affects the diaphragm. Chronic use of sleeping pills can lead to sleep apnea.

Oftentimes, losing excess body fat, eliminating allergenic foods, quitting smoking, avoiding alcohol and participating in a consistent exercise program will alleviate sleep apnea.

Additional *Winning Formulas* for those afflicted with sleep apnea include sleeping with your head slightly elevated and hydrating your nostrils with diluted MSM drops before sleep.

Aside from green tea's life-extending health benefits, consumption of green tea may be a factor in alleviating sleep-disordered breathing such as obstructive sleep apnea. Keep in mind that green tea does contain caffeine, which can affect a restful night's sleep.

Parasites are more active at night. Common symptoms of intestinal parasites include teeth grinding during sleep, nocturnal coughing in children, eye inflammation, hives, diarrhea, fever, abdominal pain and an itchy anus. Over ninety percent of all human beings have some sort of parasite. Confirmation of parasites is established through a comprehensive stool analysis.

Another reason to eliminate refined carbohydrates and sugar is because these are the perfect food source for yeast and parasites.

If a person doesn't sleep well, a liver cleansing protocol is usually in order. (Refer to Chapter 3-4 for more on the liver.) If you consistently wake up between the hours of 1:00 a.m. and 3:00 a.m., this suggests a congested, toxic liver. These are the hours when your liver is most active.

Waking up regularly between the hours of 11:00 p.m. and 1:00 a.m. may be an indication of issues with the gallbladder. Sleep disruption between the hours of 3:00 a.m. and 5:00 a.m. correlates to oxidative stress. If you're able to fall asleep, however you wake up throughout the night, this may be a symptom of hypoglycemia. If you are unable to fall asleep, consider insufficient mineral status.

If you've ever experienced insomnia or trouble falling asleep, then you know that it can be a very frustrating experience. Tossing and turning, doing mental calculations and thinking that if you just fell asleep in the next five minutes you would get this many hours of sleep, cannot only be aggravating and pointless but can actually serve to keep you awake even longer.

In acupuncture there is a point on the bottom of the feet that can help you fall asleep faster. It is located on the bottom of each foot along the centerline, about an inch north of center there is a point which lies on the kidney meridians. Pressing on this point with moderate pressure for 30-60 seconds helps to strengthen the kidneys. This point is very effective and can sometimes result is sleep as little as 30 seconds later. You can also do a general foot massage while focusing on this point to achieve the same effect.

Studies show that people who sleep more are in greater health, think more clearly, have more energy, live longer and their hearts are less strained throughout the day.

Restful sleep is a *Winning Formula* for the fountain of youth.

Winning Formulas to promote relaxation and restful sleep:

- Acupuncture treatments.

- Avoid bedtime snacks such as grains and sugars.

- Avoid caffeine. Stop all caffeine by 12:00 noon. It's very disruptive for restful sleep.

- Avoid eating anything at least two hours before bedtime.

- Avoid prescription and OTC medications.

- Check the bedroom for electromagnetic fields (EMF) which disrupt the pineal gland and affect melatonin production.

- Consider a new mattress.

- Consider helpful herbs such as Chaste tree, 120 to 480 mg.

- Consider lemon balm tincture. One dropper thirty minutes before bedtime.

- Consider magnesium, 400-600 milligrams thirty to sixty minutes before bedtime.

- Consider the herbal tranquilizer Biotics VHP (valerian, HOPS, passion flower): four capsules thirty to sixty minutes before bedtime.

- Dim the lighting; shifting the energy in your house around 8:00 p.m. Light stimulates the release of cortisol.

- Drink chamomile and lime blossom tea before bedtime.

- Drink plenty of water throughout the day (stopping by 7:00 to 8:00 p.m.). This will allow your nervous system to relax.

- Eliminate alcohol. It is very disruptive for restful sleep.

- Eliminate processed foods from your diet.

- Enjoy an Epsom salt hot bath with lavender or sandalwood ninety to 120 minutes before bedtime.

- Evaluate any prescription medications you currently take. Certain prescription and over-the-counter drugs such as steroids, decongestants and drugs for high blood pressure, depression and asthma can keep you up at night.

- Exercise regularly (not too close to bedtime).

- Get a handle on your stress.

- Have adrenals and hormones checked.

- Hide your clock to eliminate all lighting from the room. (Clock should be a minimum of five feet from your head due to the powerful electromagnetic waves it produces.)

- If diagnosed with hypertension, test for insulin resistance, heavy metal toxicity and serum vitamin D levels.

- Journal and focus on gratitude.

- Keep a notepad close to bed. If you awaken in the middle of the night with your mind racing, you can jot down your thoughts and return to sleep unworried.

- Large amounts of good quality fats help to sedate the nervous system prior to bed.

- Listen to white noise or relaxation CDs.

- Make love. Sexual activity helps to relax your body.

- Make your bedroom "sleepable." A dark, cool room is best or sleeping.

- Massage your feet, especially with warm oil, right before bed.

- Meditate. Meditation creates a calmer state and strengthens your conscious mind and will.

- Practice deep belly breathing and short breath holding exercises.

- Practice helpful yoga poses: forward folds and legs up the wall.

- Progesterone can help with sleeping although the cream may build up so high that it converts to estrogen. Sublingual seems to work better.

- Read something light or spiritual prior to bedtime. This will stimulate your parasympathetic nervous system.

- Sleep in complete darkness or as close to it as possible.

- Sleep on the proper pillow for you.

- Snack on a handful of walnuts two hours before bedtime (walnuts are a great source of tryptophan).

- Sprinkle sheets and pillow cases with lavender.

- Stop watching TV or using the computer by 8:00 p.m. The flickering light stimulates a rise in cortisol.

CHAPTER 3-2

THE POWER OF LIFESTYLE

STRESS

"Breath is aligned to both body and mind and it alone is the tool which can bring them both together, illuminating both and bringing both peace and calm."
~Thich Nhat Hanh

Stress is like dark chocolate – a little is okay and too much will kill you. An astonishing eighty to ninety percent of all illness and disease is stress-related. Stress is your reaction to your external environment, as well as your inner thoughts and feelings. Although stress is inevitable, the key is managing your stress levels.

Stress presents itself in countless forms including: sleep deprivation, marriage/relationships, poor posture, work, negative thoughts, dieting, kids, poor food choices, food allergies, injuries, lack of exercise, noise pollution, electromagnetic waves (computer, television, alarm clocks, cell phones and microwave oven), dehydration, finances, crowds, digestive distress (immune system), chemical, environmental, travel, psycho-spiritual stress, substance abuse and imbalanced hormones.

From this lengthy list you can see how stress is the number one cause of disease. How destructive can stress be for your body?

Stress is a precursor to cancer. Stress, anger and general emotional imbalance can lead to an acidic environment in your body. Human beings are hard-wired. Your system does not know the difference from various stressors. Stress can manifest as perceived, real or imagined stress.

According to research in the *American Journal of Public Health*, "low back pain can have its roots in stress experienced much earlier in life. Psychological stress at age twenty-three increases the likelihood of low back pain at age thirty-three."

Stress affects your brain by releasing powerful chemicals called neurotransmitters, such as dopamine, norepinephrine, epinephrine or adrenaline. The connecting factor among physical, emotional and mental stressors occurs in an area of your brain known as the HPA axis consisting of the pituitary, adrenals and hypothalamus. The HPA axis releases growth hormone (GH) and cortisol. Chronic stress over time eventually shrinks the hypothalamus. The hypothalamus is found above the brain stem and controls body temperature, fatigue, hunger, thirst, anger and circadian cycles.

Your nervous system registers every stressful event. It sends chemical and electrical impulses to every tissue, cell and organ of your body. Symptoms of stress may appear in your body as a headache, digestive issues, heart palpitations, pain, clammy palms or nausea. Research has shown that prolonged episodes of stress actually create changes to your tissue and cause organ dysfunction.

The organs that suffer the most from stress are your stomach and pancreas. Individuals diagnosed with autoimmune diseases, such as chronic fatigue syndrome or fibromyalgia, have repeatedly experienced an overwhelming accumulation of stressful events – psychologically, physically or emotionally – in their lives.

Traditional Chinese Medicine and acupuncture reveal:

- Stress in the form of anger decreases the liver's ability to filter, cleanse and circulate blood.
- Stress in the form of fear affects the kidneys.
- Stress in the form of frustration affects the gallbladder.
- Stress in the form of grief damages the lungs leading to respiratory infections.
- Stress, in the form of worry, creates digestive system dysfunction.

If a woman experiences excessive stress and becomes pregnant two years later, her fetus is affected. If you're planning to have a child, BOTH sexes should be tested for heavy metal toxicity. Approximately thirty percent of females have enough mercury in their systems to put a fetus at risk.

The adverse affects of heavy metals, including arsenic, cadmium, lead and mercury, are of great concern to the general public and the medical community.

Mercury accumulation is possible from dental amalgam fillings, inks used by various printers and tattooists, several cosmetics, vaccines, various plastics and consumption of contaminated fish.

Elevated levels of mercury have been linked to autism, attention-deficit disorder, cognitive decline, hypertension, breast cancer, infertility and Multiple Sclerosis. Mercury poisoning may cause neurological, gastrointestinal, immune and mental disorders.

Recent studies have shown that lead exposure can lead to higher rates of Parkinson's disease and cognitive decline in adults, as well as lower IQ and learning difficulties in children. Lead exposure is associated with ADD and ADHD, ringing in the ears, anti-social behavior, diminished ability to concentrate, cognitive dysfunction and a lowered functioning immune system. Most chocolate is high in lead.

Cadmium has estrogenic activity and is associated with increased risk for osteoporosis, kidney damage and cancer.

Arsenic, a known carcinogen, is present in many municipal and private water supplies and can increase the risk for diabetes.

Aluminum, the most abundant metal, has been linked with Alzheimer's disease, amyotrophic lateral sclerosis, also known as ALS or Lou Gehrig's disease, as well as other neurological disorders and cognitive problems. Excess aluminum comes from deodorants, antacids, many OTC drugs, table salt and aluminum cookware and foil.

Another stressor we seldom consider is electromagnetic stress. Electromagnetic stress is emitted from electrical devices, mobile phones, fluorescent lighting, televisions, microwave ovens and computers. Affected individuals frequently complain of headaches and fatigue. Some claim to receive a mild shock when touching metal objects.

Electromagnetic stress can cause a vast range of side effects, from mild to severe, including:

- Allergies
- An inability to relax or get restful sleep
- Depression
- Headaches
- Illnesses caused by a weakened immune system
- Reduced testosterone levels
- Stress related illness, such as heart-attacks
- Tinnitus (continuous ringing in the ears)

Studies on the effects of exposure to electromagnetic fields are ongoing. A study of cancer cells indicated that the "cells grow over twenty times the normal rate when exposed to electromagnetic fields." In yet another study, "changes were produced in the cerebellums of newborn animals whose parents were exposed to electromagnetic stress." The cerebellum is a portion of the brain responsible for coordination of movement and balance.

Microwave ovens are a major source of electromagnetic stress. Foods cooked in a microwave oven cause suppression of your immune system. Consuming microwaved foods change your cellular polarity (from clockwise to counterclockwise) causing damage to your cellular structure. With repeated exposure, there is an increase in symptoms, such as fatigue, headaches, memory loss, irritability, sleeping problems and deep tissue burns.

Additional damaging effects caused from eating food cooked in a microwave oven:

- Eating microwaved foods cause an increase in the number of cancer cells in your blood. Microwaved foods bring about cancerous stomach and intestinal tumors.
- Microwaved food alters or completely shuts down hormone production. Microwaved food increases total cholesterol.
- Microwaving vegetables destroy ninety-seven percent of their flavonoids. Boiling destroys sixty-six percent and steaming produces only minimal loss.

Stress has a negative impact on your libido. When one begins to exhibit stress-related symptoms (such as a decreased sex drive) one may have been exhibiting these symptoms for such a period of time that they have begun to accept them as normal.

There are many other causes of sexual dysfunction or a low sex drive. Some of the most common causes are cardiovascular, renal, nutritional, hormonal, emotional, neurological, pharmacological and environmental toxins.

The best thing to try to improve one's sex life is to reduce stress levels. Often just by trying things like meditation, exercise, dance, laughter, massage and hobbies, stress levels can be effectively reduced and all aspects of life (including intimacy) can become much more enjoyable.

Mind-body activities such as yoga, tai chi, breathing exercises, hypnosis and meditation are great stress-busters. Meditation doesn't require formal training or education. Its purpose is to clear your mind so you can calmly think about what's causing your stress and regain a sense of peace.

Breathe! The average person breathes 20,000 breaths daily. If you're stressed out or you tend to breathe from your chest versus your diaphragm, your breathing patterns increase up to 40,000 breaths per day. Your diaphragm is a large muscle located between your chest and abdomen (under the ribs). Deep, full breaths create a healthy, balanced nervous system. When you breathe using your diaphragm, the belly expands as you inhale. The breathing is performed through your nose with your neck, chest and shoulders completely relaxed. As you exhale, focus on drawing your navel toward your spine by contracting your lower abdominal muscles. Take a moment right now to take in a few diaphragmatic breaths. Notice the subtle changes within.

Attention to your breathing habits can actually change your cellular physiology. Doing so energizes your body, improving your ability to focus and concentrate. Full, deep breathing throughout the day can eliminate acid buildup as well as reduce physiological and mental-emotional stress. Your cells use oxygen to convert glucose into energy called adenosine triphosphate (ATP). Cells begin to die and energy cannot be sufficiently produced without sufficient oxygen. Deep breathing revitalizes and energizes every cell.

In addition to strengthening your diaphragm muscle, diaphragmatic breathing stimulates your parasympathetic nervous system creating a sense of relaxation and calm.

Deep, full breathing stimulates your immune system, improves digestion and cleanses your organs. Your breathing patterns provide positive benefits on all levels – physically, mentally, emotionally and spiritually.

Diaphragmatic breathing delivers oxygen to your tissues and cells assisting in the removal of toxins from your body. As you take deeper breaths, your body removes toxins from your system by blowing off carbon dioxide, thereby lessening the carbonic acid in the blood. Deep breathing increases lymphatic circulation and normalizes blood pressure.

Practice this *Winning Formula* breathing pattern for three to five minutes daily: breathe in to the count of four, hold two counts, exhale to the count of eight and hold two counts before you inhale.

Meditation helps manage your overall stress levels. Solitude and meditation are effective in preventing obesity and degenerative illness. Urban living tends to over-stimulate your senses. Taking the time for yourself may seem impossible when faced with a stressful situation, however it is important to remain centered in the midst of a storm. Your center is a place that is naturally joyful and at peace. Connecting with any natural environment such as a park, beach or mountains on a regular basis allows you to connect with Mother Nature. Your ability to communicate with God is enhanced when you're in a peaceful, natural environment away from artificial noises.

What you do, how you live and the choices you make in your twenties and thirties begin to surface in your forties. Your choices made today directly impact your state of balance tomorrow. Balance is a state of non-stress – a feeling. You know when you're there.

We all respond differently to stressful events because of our personal interpretation and the various resources and skills to deal or manage with the situation. Some situations which are not negative may still be perceived as stressful. This is because we think we are not completely prepared to cope with them effectively. It is important to learn that what matters more than the event itself is usually our thoughts about the event when we are trying to manage stress. How you see that stressful event will be the largest single factor that impacts on your physical and mental health. Your interpretation of events and challenges in life may decide whether they are invigorating or harmful for you.

How do you alleviate, deal with, manage or diminish stress in your life?

- Be aware.
- Choose and practice activities that create balance.
- Implement *Winning Formulas* for stress reduction from the following list.

Winning Formulas for stress reduction:

- Animals and pets
- Appropriate exercise
- Artwork
- Biofeedback
- Chiropractic adjustments for correct alignment of the spine
- Connect with nature
- Diaphragmatic breathing

- Eliminate cooking foods in the microwave oven
- Extending love and kindness to self and others
- Hobbies
- Hot baths with Epsom or Celtic sea salts and essential oils
- Hypnosis
- Journaling
- Laughing, watching a comedy

- Listening to music, especially classical
- Massage
- Meditation
- Minimize cell phone use
- Playing a musical instrument
- Positive thoughts and mental attitude

- Postural awareness
- Prayer
- Quality nutrition
- Reading inspirational books
- Remove electrical devices from bedroom
- Repeating a manta: word or phrase that has meaning to you

- Rest and restful sleep
- Set boundaries
- Sex
- Simplify your to-do list; prioritize
- Singing
- Solitude and nature
- Stretching
- Support groups

- Surround yourself with positive, like-minded people
- Thoughts of love, compassion and gratitude
- Volunteering
- Walking
- Water/ocean
- Yoga, Tai Chi and/or Qi Gong

CHAPTER 3-3

THE POWER OF LIFESTYLE

THOUGHTS AND ATTITUDE

"You become great by thinking great thoughts and by backing those thoughts with your words, energy, emotions and actions. Encourage yourself to leave behind negative and uphold positive, uplifting ideas with your speech. This is how your dreams will be able to manifest from the inside out."
~Carol Tuttle

Your thoughts are the very first thing turned on when you awake. Everything starts with a thought. All thoughts are stored in your subconscious, as well as your physical body. Negative, toxic thoughts may manifest as physical pain, bad attitudes and eventually, disease. Your attitude and emotional state are critical in fighting disease. Physical congestion may show up as blocked arteries or a messy office. Emotional congestion may present itself as sustained grief. When you are congested spiritually, this may signify that you are unable to forgive yourself for past mistakes.

Your thoughts and emotions determine the direction your life is heading toward. Reflect on your life. Doing so often reveals your deeper beliefs.

It's as though life is a mirror reflecting back at you what you think about. Feelings of frustration and irritation create an unfulfilled life of discontent and unhappiness. The more joy-filled you are the more you create and fulfill your purpose and destiny.

You have the power to change your negative thoughts to positive thoughts through desire, determination, consistency, self-hypnosis, prayer or affirmations. You are the "creator" of your life. Your mind can be your best friend or worst enemy depending what you choose to think about. Your mind is much more powerful than your feelings.

Your emotions can flow in the direction of positive, solution-based thoughts or in the direction of negative, conflict and crisis-type thoughts. Engaging a positive thought process is a **Winning Formula** for overall health. Your emotions determine the state of your autonomic nervous system. When you are upset, your sympathetic nervous system responds by releasing stress hormones, which further enhance a catabolic (muscle loss) environment in your body. Happiness and calm activates your parasympathetic nervous system. This content state stimulates the release of anabolic (muscle growth) hormones, thus boosting your immune system and stimulating your body's ability to recover.

Everything you are creating in your life is a reflection of what you've allowed yourself and others to plant within you.

The Universal Law of Vibration explains that each thought is a vibration. This means everything is moving, swinging and dancing, including your thoughts, whether you can see the movement or not.

Accept your emotions without the need to over analyze, control or fix them as this creates more tension which adds to more stress. It also creates inner struggle. On a physical level, emotions are felt throughout your body as molecules called neuropeptides which attach themselves onto cellular receptors. When an emotion is felt, but not expressed, these molecules of emotion get stuck in your system seeking a way out. Expression of the emotion and ownership of the experience is required without fixing, doing or psychoanalyzing.

Every time you allow another person to trigger emotions of fear, anger, grief or sadness you give them permission to disconnect your soul with your Higher Power. When you respond to positive stimuli such as joy, happiness and peace, you are creating a vibrational agreement with it.

People who consistently have thoughts of negativity tend to be destructive to themselves and to those around them. Negative thoughts are damaging to the person thinking them, as well as to those who resonate with them.

Individuals who choose to live with a positive mind-set create hope. They are valuable to themselves as well as those around them. Take charge of your life by taking charge of your thoughts.

You can completely transform your life by changing the way you think. Your thoughts transmit an invisible energy that affects your mental and physical well-being.

You can alter your home or work environment to encourage positive habits. If a certain activity or a person drains you of energy, do what you can to eliminate that activity or person from your life. Instead, surround yourself with people who love and support you. Choose to live your life around the job, people and activities that fulfill you and make you feel good.

You are in control of every thought. *Winning Formula* thoughts include: love, compassion, joy, appreciation, contentment, gratitude and prosperity.

Ultimately, it is your responsibility. The choices you make move you closer or further away from your deserved joy, purpose and happiness. Focus on positive outcomes and desired actions.

Your subconscious belief system is extremely powerful. Those beliefs create your perception and outlook on life. You can change these deep-rooted beliefs by altering your thoughts. Changing your thinking can change your brain's neurochemistry. Neurons that fire together wire together. Every thought, positive or negative, causes neurons to stimulate the release of neurotransmitters and hormones. What you concentrate on expands. Your *Winning Formula* is to focus on an "attitude of gratitude."

In her book, "Molecules of Emotion," Candace Pert states the following: *"We must take responsibility for the way we feel. The notion that others can make us feel good or bad is untrue. Consciously, or more frequently unconsciously, we are choosing how we feel at every single moment. The external world is in so many ways a mirror of our beliefs and expectations. Why we feel the way we feel is the result of the symphony and harmony of our own molecules of emotion that affect every aspect of our physiology, producing blissful good health or miserable disease."*

There is no solution outside of you to experience bliss, health or happiness. You are the solution and will be guided to what you need intuitively once you connect with your emotions.

One of my favorite authors, Louise Hay, writes in her book *Heal Your Body,* how physical disease originates from your mental and emotional thought process.

Louise teaches: *"The mental thought patterns that cause the most disease in the body are criticism, resentment, anger and guilt. Your physical being is your Creator's last effort in communicating to you that something is seriously wrong. Louise writes that criticism often leads to arthritis. Anger shows up as things that burn, boil and infect the body. Resentments lead to cancer and tumors. Guilt always seeks punishment and leads to pain."*

119

In order to move forward and live a joy-filled life, it's essential that you release anything that no longer serves you. Doing so allows space for positive and beneficial changes to present themselves. Energize the ideas you wish to manifest instead of directing all your thought and energy into what you do not want. Focus on what you want. Get emotionally charged. Imagine, visualize and act as though you already have all you desire.

Affirmations are positive statements that can be used to create change. Affirmations manifest your dreams and desires into reality. These positive statements focus your consciousness on your power to create and have what you want. Affirmations create change in how you think about yourself and your health.

Since your subconscious mind doesn't know the difference between a real or imagined idea, your mind responds to whatever suggestions you feed it.

Affirmations can be thought of as a tool you use to free yourself from thoughts that no longer serve you in a positive light. By repeating a positive affirmation when a self-defeating negative thought enters your mind, you reprogram your mind. Eventually, the old, negative thought patterns will lose their emotional charge and stop altogether. The words "I AM" are two of the most powerful words to verbalize in creating what you want.

Choose from the *Winning Formula* affirmations listed below or create your own. Your affirmations should be positive and attainable.

Examples of *Winning Formula* affirmations may include:
• God loves me and I love myself.
• I am a valuable person in charge of my destiny.
• I am allowing myself permission to attract love, prosperity and health.
• I am an exceptional human being.
• I am attracting like-minded people to work with.
• I am completely secure and love who I am physically, emotionally and spiritually.
• I am creating more of what I want in easy ways.
• I am deserving of a healthy, fit body and healthy lifestyle.
• I am financially independent.
• I am grateful for my health.
• I am living a balanced life that fulfills me on all levels.
• I am losing weight easily.
• I am magnetic to my Higher good.
• I am open, mind and heart, to new, creative experiences.
• I am radiantly healthy in body, mind and spirit.

- I am ready to be healed, calmed and empowered.
- I am successful in life and love.
- I am the key to peace.
- I am the source of my abundance and prosperity.
- I am willing to release anything that is not for my higher good.
- I am worthy of real love. I deserve to be loved by a healthy, emotionally available person.
- I attract only healthy, win-win relationships that benefit me on all levels.
- I choose to associate with people of high integrity.
- I commit to expressing appreciation to those I love.
- I have faith in myself.
- I love my body unconditionally.
- I stand in my power.

Affirmations can be used in any area of your life. Choose one or two affirmations daily. Memorize and repeat your affirmations throughout the day. When a negative thought enters your mind, cancel that thought. Replace it with a *Winning Formula* affirmation listed above or create one of your own.

Expressing gratitude regularly has been linked to better health and well-being. Look for things and people to appreciate. A Grateful Log is an invaluable **Winning Formula** to include in your daily routine. At the end of each day, write down five things for which you are grateful. You can log this in a spiral notebook.

Surround yourself with like-minded people. You are the average of the five people you spend the most time with. Dissolving relationships that are no longer serving you in a positive manner will always lead to healing. All endings are inexorably tied to new beginnings.

Set firm boundaries. The minute you consent to being around someone with a lower, negative vibration, you lose your joy, leaving yourself wide open to attract the outcome of their beliefs and moods. You can send positive, loving thoughts and energy to someone who is vibrating from negative emotions. When your mind is filled with light, there is no room for darkness. When you maintain a higher energy around a 'doom-and-gloom' person, you will know that you're in alignment with your desires, dreams and destiny.

Ask yourself: "Does this person make me feel good?" Make a list of the people you associate with. If you could put a plus (+) or minus (–) in front of their names, how many would have pluses?

Negative energy individuals have an enormous influence on you if you continue to surround yourselves with them. The backbone of your happiness rests on your relationships and the growth and development of your sense of purpose. Eliminate draining people, environments, activities and things from your life.

Choose what energizes you. Learn to feel the energy of a situation, place or person. As your energy changes, you'll want different energy around you. If something feels right, you feel in harmony mentally, spiritually and emotionally. Listen to your body and emotions. Be attentive to what you need. This could be a walk in nature, repeating a prayer, the voice of a friend, a book or poem that speaks to your soul or your favorite music. You are here to feel joy and absorb all of life's beauty.

Focus on positive outcomes and desired actions. Positive emotional states are liked to prolonged life expectancy. The key *Winning Formula* to remember is that your thoughts always create your reality. You are in charge of your thoughts.

NEVER SURRENDER YOUR JOY.

CHAPTER 3-4

THE POWER OF LIFESTYLE

HEALTHY HORMONAL BALANCE

"We spend more, but have less; we buy more, but enjoy it less. We have bigger houses and smaller families; more conveniences, but less time; we have more degrees, but less sense; more knowledge, but less judgment; more experts, but more problems; more medicine, but less wellness. We've added years to life, not life to years."
~Jason Day

Every function of your body is controlled by your hormones. All of your glands are connected to each other. Hormones deliver messages to your cells regarding your metabolism. The endocrine system controls much of your body's regulating hormones, your body's pH, body temperature and chemicals in your bloodstream, all of which are delicately balanced and vulnerable if altered for a significant length of time. Your hormones affect your moods, as well as your thoughts. When your hormones are balanced, you feel fabulous. When they're out of balance, you experience exhaustion, depression, lowered immunity, decreased libido and increased body fat.

Conditions associated with imbalanced hormones:

- Arthritis
- Asthma
- Autoimmune Disorders
- Cancer
- Chronic Fatigue Syndrome

- Depression
- Diabetes
- Fibromyalgia
- Heart disease
- Hypertension

- Hypotension
- Immune system diseases
- Inflammation
- Infertility
- Osteoporosis
- Thyroid problems

Hormones such as insulin, cortisol, epinephrine, as well as estrogen, progesterone, DHEA, testosterone, melatonin and human growth hormone begin to decline as we age. Hormones do not act independently. Hormones work in synergy. As hormones decline, so do other functions, such as enzyme activity and detoxification performance.

In order for hormones to function properly, fat is a mandatory component! Cholesterol is the precursor to sex hormones in your body. Pregnenolone, known as the mother hormone, is a precursor to progesterone, cortisol, DHEA, estrogen and testosterone. DHEA is one of the most abundant hormones in the body. Under stressful conditions, these hormones are often inhibited. Hormonal disruption is a factor to consider for lacking libido.

In addition, when your body is stressed, your adrenal glands release corticosteroids. Just five minutes of anger increase your cortisol levels for six hours! Cortisol's job is to restore peace and calmness to the body and mind, enabling us to deal with the stressful situation with a level head. Cortisol regulates blood pressure and cardiovascular function as well as the body's use of proteins, carbohydrates and fats.

Co-factors for all hormones include vitamins A and B-6, zinc and magnesium. There are many factors to consider for hormonal balance. Aside from aging, as mentioned above, stress is a major culprit for hormonal imbalances.

High cortisol levels are linked to low thyroid function. Cortisol is the number one pro-aging hormone. Lupus, osteoporosis, fibromyalgia, sugar or salt cravings, digestive problems and allergies may indicate high cortisol. Other symptoms are feeling overly stressed, confusion, skin problems, respiratory difficulties, difficulty concentrating and indifference toward sex.

If your cortisol levels are elevated, consider testing for parasites. Parasites cause long-term, low level inflammation that place demands on your adrenal glands to constantly secrete higher levels of cortisol over the years. Parasites tend to become more active at night, stimulating your adrenals to elevate your cortisol levels. Cortisol should be declining at the end of the day. Parasites are confirmed via stool testing. A combination of anti-parasitic supplements will kill these bugs. (See Resources.)

Hypothyroidism is epidemic in our society, as well as iodine deficiency. The thyroid is responsible for your metabolism.

Children of hypothyroid mothers were found to have abnormal visual processing, lower IQ levels, deficits in attention, as well as in sensorimotor skills and memory. Mild hypothyroidism in pregnant women secondary to iodine deficiency is associated with lower IQ and cognitive deficits in their children. It is recommended that all women have a complete thyroid panel taken prior to becoming pregnant, and again once their baby is born.

Indications of an underactive thyroid may include:

- Achy joints
- Anemia
- Brittle nails
- Cold hands and feet
- Constipation
- Dry skin
- Edema
- Frequent infections
- Goiter
- Hair loss
- Hoarse voice
- Hypertension
- Hypotension
- Insomnia
- Loss of or lack of libido
- Macroglossia (bulging eyes)
- Poor eyebrow growth (especially the outer third)
- Puffy face
- Sluggish reflexes (Achilles tendon)
- Tender Achilles tendon (when palpated at the insertion)
- Tinnitus (ringing in ears)

Scientific studies showed a sluggish thyroid system was directly related to increased mortality, fatal heart disease, disturbed heart rhythms, elevated blood pressure, elevated cholesterol, lack of coordination, an increased risk of breast cancer, mood problems, glaucoma and Alzheimer's risk.

Here's an easy *Winning Formula* to assess the function of your thyroid for hypothyroidism in the privacy of your home. Take your first morning temperature (orally). Monitor your temperature for five consecutive days. Total the number. Divide by five for an average temperature. If your average temperature is lower than 97.8 this may indicate:

- Adrenal or pituitary deficiencies
- An underactive thyroid
- Fertility issues
- Starvation

Natural *Winning Formula* thyroid boosters include: L-tyrosine, iodine, magnesium, coconut oil, eliminating aspartame, trans fats, soy and gluten, castor oil packs three times weekly and yoga poses such as shoulder stand, fish, plow and the bridge.

It is an essential *Winning Formula* to have adequate levels of iodine for a healthy functioning thyroid gland.

Not only is iodine crucial to thyroid health it is a *Winning Formula* for optimal immune health. Iodine contains potent anti-bacterial, anti-parasitic, anti-viral and anti-cancer properties.

Hypothyroidism often goes hand in hand with an iodine deficiency. Approximately sixty percent of total iodine is stored in your thyroid gland. Iodine is concentrated in the ovaries, breast and prostate tissue. The breasts and ovaries will uptake iodine at about the same rate as the thyroid. There is a direct association with iodine deficiency and increased risk for prostate, endometrial, ovarian and breast cancers. Iodine deficiency will result in dysfunction in one or all of these areas. The male also shares iodine with other organs, although at a rate less than that of the female breast and ovary. It becomes obvious why there are more females than males with hypothyroidism.

Treatment of thyroid hypo function without iodine increases the rate of fibroids and breast cancer. If you are being treated with thyroid hormone while your body is deficient in iodine, the thyroid hormone may exacerbate the iodine deficiency. Initially, you may feel better on thyroid hormones, however the iodine deficiency may actually worsen the thyroid condition, even though you are taking prescribed hormones.

David Brownstein, MD explains in his book, *Iodine, Why You Need It, Why You Can't Live Without It*, your thyroid requires iodine to regulate your metabolism and to produce hormones. Dr. Brownstein has found that proper supplementation with iodine cures or improves an underactive thyroid.

Fish is a concentrated food source of iodine. Other sources of iodine include Celtic sea salt and sea vegetables, such as kelp and seaweed, and plants grown in iodine-rich soil.

Iodine supplementation is a healing *Winning Formula* for many other conditions including breast, ovarian and prostate diseases, migraine headaches, cystic breasts, ADD, infertility and vaginal infections. Some individuals are able to discontinue their thyroid hormone completely and take only iodine once their iodine levels are within optimal range. Work with a qualified health practitioner to assess your iodine levels. Supplementing with the proper dosage is extremely important, as too much iodine is also problematic.

Iodine deficiency is a worldwide problem. Seventy-two percent of the world's population is affected by iodine deficiency. Vegetarians are usually deficient in iodine. Between 1971 and 2000, the National Health and Nutrition survey showed iodine levels declined fifty percent in the United States. In the 1960s, iodine was added to bakery products as an anti-caking agent. In the 1970s, bromine was substituted for iodine due to misinformation about iodine. Bromine is added to many soft drinks as brominated vegetable oil. You'll find it in Mountain Dew, Amp Energy drinks and some Gatorade products.

Read the list of ingredients on every product!

Bromine is a toxic substance with no known value for your body. Bromine is an antibacterial agent for pools and hot tubs, a fumigant for agriculture, termites and other pests. Bromine interferes with iodine utilization in your body. It disturbs the function of your thyroid, testes and adrenals.

Symptoms of iodine deficiency include: goiter, infertility, mental impairment, ADD, as well as increased risk of breast, prostate, endometrial, ovarian and other cancers.

It is especially important for individuals with an underactive thyroid to eliminate all plastics, mercury, soy and fluoridated products. Buy fluoride-free toothpaste.

Mercury toxicity may diminish thyroid function because it displaces the trace mineral, selenium. Selenium is involved in conversion of thyroid hormones T4 to T3.

If you have mercury amalgam fillings, consider removing them. Mercury released from fillings builds up in the brain, pituitary, adrenals and other parts of the body. Mercury amalgam fillings should be removed **only** by dentists with experience using the International Academy of Oral Medicine and Toxicology (IAOMT) mercury amalgam removal protocol.

A recent study published in the *Journal of Orthomolecular Medicine* related to the proper removal of mercury amalgam fillings from 118 subjects showed an elimination or reduction of eighty percent of the classic mercury poisoning symptoms.

In many cases, it took six to twelve months after mercury amalgam removal for the symptoms to disappear. Smaller, coldwater fish such as sardines, anchovies, wild salmon and halibut contain less mercury. Other 'lower-mercury' fish include flounder, catfish, perch, herring, whitefish, mahi, cod and pollock.

Attention to adrenal health and balanced insulin levels should not be overlooked when addressing hypothyroid disorders.

Signs of overtaxed adrenal glands are exhaustion, weight gain, hair falling out, irritability and the most tell-tale sign, skin rashes and acne. Other symptoms include: arthritic tendencies, inflammation, chronic low back pain, heartburn, blood sugar imbalances, reduced thyroid, chronic infections and colds, low serotonin levels, a "need" to wear sunglasses, low libido, sleep disruption, poor concentration and/or memory, tending to be a "night" person, medial knee pain and sugar and/or salt cravings.

Adrenal dysfunction slows down metabolism and contributes to increased body fat storage, especially around the midsection. Adrenal fatigue and adrenal exhaustion affects sixty percent of the population. Dr. James Wilson explains this quite brilliantly in his book, *Adrenal Fatigue, The 21st Century Stress Syndrome*. Adrenal fatigue is caused by prolonged stress (emotional, physical, electromagnetic or psychological), eating foods you're sensitive to, exposure to toxins, skipping meals and blood sugar imbalances, chronic use of stimulants and insufficient rest and relaxation.

Saliva testing is the most reliable diagnosis of adrenal fatigue. Saliva samples are taken four times in one day to determine basic cortisol rhythms. An organic diet with adequate protein will help to restore adrenal health and maintain blood sugar stability. Various vitamins, glandulars and herbs assist in recovery for your adrenals. Stress management is crucial to restore adrenal health. Include brisk walking and avoid high-intensity cardiovascular exercise.

Selective serotonin reuptake inhibitors (SSRIs) are a class of antidepressant medications used in the treatment of depression, anxiety disorders and some personality disorders. SSRIs focus on various neurotransmitters of the brain, particularly serotonin.

Neurotransmitters such as serotonin and dopamine create feelings of motivation and relaxation. Sleep, diet and exercise strongly influence serotonin and dopamine. Ninety percent of serotonin is produced in your gastrointestinal tract. SSRIs suppress cortisol by up to seventy percent. Extended use of SSRIs will inhibit your natural production of serotonin. The most common side effects when taking SSRIs include: headache, nausea, drowsiness, weight/appetite fluctuations as well as increased feelings of anxiety or depression. A recent Canadian study found "patients prescribed SSRI antidepressants were five times more likely to commit suicide or have suicidal thoughts and behavior." On top of that, these drugs destroy your sex drive!

All drugs have side effects.

In a seminar taught by Charles Poliquin, he discussed an interesting point regarding body piercings. Charles stated that "body piercings disrupt all hormones, especially piercings on the midline, such as the belly button or lips. Piercings on the midline of the body also cause fertility issues. These energy meridians are over-stimulated by the piercings."

Human growth hormone (HGH) is secreted while you sleep and during resistance exercise. HGH is advertised as the "anti-aging" hormone. It helps repair tissue and promotes growth. Optimal secretion depends on deep, restful sleep for eight hours. HGH is also dependent on the availability of amino acids which is supplied from the protein you eat. Alcohol suppresses HGH, is estrogenic and causes feminine characteristics in men. Although HGH injections are advertised as the "fountain of youth," one must be cautious with HGH injections. Discuss the pros and cons with your natural health practitioner. Someone who has been injecting HGH and who has an unknown space-occupying lesion or tumor will only exacerbate this condition. There are less harmful, more natural methods to increase your levels of growth hormone.

The male version of menopause is known as andropause. Men experience a gradual decline in testicular function, as well as testosterone production. Testosterone production drops about fifty percent between the ages of forty and seventy. Lower testosterone levels in men often indicate a zinc deficiency.

By the time a man reaches his mid-fifties, symptoms of andropause are noticeable, although symptoms may appear earlier. Aging is the number one cause of andropause and declining testosterone levels. However, other factors include: stress, medical conditions such as diabetes, prior use of steroids, mental illness, poor diet, medications, excessive alcohol consumption and obesity.

Testosterone is an anabolic steroid that builds strong bones and muscles. It's critical for a strong, functioning heart. Testosterone does much more than fuel your libido. Testosterone keeps your brain operating at peak performance. Testosterone provides powerful anti-aging effects for women. It works with estrogen to keep skin supple, increase bone mineral density, boost mood and increase the ability to handle stress.

Symptoms of testosterone deficiency include low libido, depression, lack of motivation, low energy, reduced muscle and bone mass, hair loss and memory impairment. Low testosterone levels put your at risk for Alzheimer's disease, heart attack, stroke and many other health problems.

Aside from aging, testosterone disruption may be related to chemicals in the environment, pollution and electromagnetic stressors such as cell phones, computers, microwave ovens and television. The more television one watches the less testosterone they usually have. Men who wear their cell phones on vibrate on their hips can show up to a thirty percent decrease in testosterone.

Progesterone has a calming effect in the body. It builds bone, and is a natural diuretic and fat burner. It restores proper cellular oxygen levels, improves vascular tone, normalizes blood clotting, and prevents cyclical migraines and arterial plaque. Progesterone helps balance the actions of estrogen and acts with estrogen and testosterone to prevent cancer and other degenerative diseases. A low level of progesterone results in irritability, anxiety, obsessive behaviors, weight gain, itching, sweating, digestive problems, flatulence, bloating and loss of memory.

Estrogen is a broad category with three primary members, estradiol, estrone, and estriol. Estradiol is produced in the ovaries by the aromatization process during which the androgen hormone, androstenedione, is converted to estrone, which is then converted to estradiol. Smaller amounts of estradiol are produced by the adrenal cortex, brain and arterial walls. Testosterone can also be converted to estradiol in the body. Estrogen dominance affects men and women, alike. Estrogen dominance is determined by various factors such as genetics, lifestyle and the environment. The flabby stomach and enlarged breasts of middle aged men are a signal that their estrogen levels are too high. Many men over the age of fifty have estrogen levels that are higher than those of women over fifty.

Dr. Harry Eidenier, Jr., Ph.D. quotes: *"We are swimming in a sea of estrogen."*

Symptoms of estrogen dominance:

- Cervical dysplasia
- Decreased libido
- Difficulty with conception
- Endometriosis
- Fibrocystic or painful breasts
- Fluid retention and weight gain
- Gynecomastia (male breast growth)
- PMS, cramps, bloating
- Prostate, testes, ovarian, uterine and breast cancers
- Uterine fibroids

Estrogen dominance may be revealed through caliper skin fold measurements and hormonal lab testing. Test results may indicate high estrogen and low testosterone. This applies to males as well as females. High estrogen and low testosterone levels may be affected by aromatase enzyme.

Aromatase is found in estrogen-producing cells in the adrenal glands, ovaries, placenta, testicles, adipose or fat tissue and the brain.

Aromatization happens when androgens (testosterone) convert to estrogens (estrodial). Aging increases aromatase activity.

Liver enzyme activity and poor detoxification of estrogens are other factors to address. Alcohol is often the main culprit here, although it could be marijuana. A weight management program may be very helpful in reducing aromatase activity and facilitating estrogen metabolism and excretion.

Excess estrogens in the body may lead to aromatization as well as estrogen-dominant health issues such as PMS, endometriosis, fibroids and breast cancer. In males estrogen dominance may reveal as prostate conditions, as well as gynecomastia, a hormonal-induced growth in men's breasts tissue. This creates fatty areas or enlargement of the breast tissue.

Surgical clinics surveyed by *The Sunday Times* in Britain reported a sharp upsurge in the numbers of men seeking breast reduction surgery. Hormones in the water are blamed for a doubling of cases in just one year of gynecomastia.

Two major sources of exogenous estrogens are oral contraceptives and hormone replacement therapy. Another major source is environmental toxins that are structurally similar to estrogen and have the ability to mimic harmful estrogens in your body.

Estrogen precursors and xenoestrogens include aromatic hydrocarbons and organochlorines found in pesticides, herbicides, refrigerants, cookware with Teflon coating, industrial solvents and plastics.

Furthermore, the synthetic hormones used to fatten livestock and promote milk production may be unknowingly ingested when consuming non-organic meat and milk products, thereby increasing your exposure to environmental estrogens. This is one more reason to choose organic foods over non-organic.

The products you rub or massage into your skin may contribute to hormonal disruption. Your skin is the most absorbable organ in your body. Whatever you put on your skin is absorbed through your bloodstream. Would it surprise you to find out that more than a third of personal care products contain ingredients linked to hormonal disruption and cancer? This includes most sunscreens.

Eliminate perfumes, lotions and colognes as the majority of these products contain parabens and synthetic chemicals. You'll also find synthetic chemicals and parabens in cosmetics, deodorants, soaps and shampoos.

Studies have shown that parabens mimic the activity of estrogen. This is associated with certain forms of breast cancer, diminished muscle mass, unwanted body fat and male gynecomastia (breast growth).

The EPA has linked methyl parabens to metabolic, developmental, hormonal and neurological disorders, as well as various cancers.

Choose instead to use natural cleaning products and natural brands of personal care products. It is important to remember that everything you slather onto your skin and scalp goes directly into your bloodstream. ***Winning Formula*** – make sure you read the list of ingredients.

Aside from implementing lifestyle changes, there are various nutrients that effectively inhibit aromatase and reduce estrogen load by supporting preferred pathways of estrogen metabolism and detoxification.

Natural ***Winning Formula*** nutrients to reduce estrogen and inhibit aromatase activity include:

- B vitamins
- Calcium D-glucarate
- Chrysin
- DIM
- Green tea
- Indole-3-carbinol
- Limonene
- Magnesium (See Chapter 5-5.)
- Probiotics (See Chapter 5-4.)
- Resveratrol
- Zinc

The influences of these nutrients on estrogen metabolism may have profound significance for estrogen dominant diseases.

Factors that raise estrogen levels include:

- Carbohydrate intolerance and insulin resistance. This affects your adrenals and all other major hormones. (The hormone you have the most control over is insulin. This is controlled through your diet. Hormones do not act independently.)
- Liver function changes as well as liver stressors. Unresolved anger and resentments are stored in this organ.
- Obesity – High estrogen is present in most obese people of all ages. Obesity increases endogenous estrogen production in the fat tissue where the enzyme aromatase converts androgen hormones into estrogen. Obesity in males equals twenty-five percent body fat or greater. Obesity in females equals thirty percent body fat or greater.
- Overuse of alcohol or marijuana.
- Prescription drug side effects – especially diuretics and liver activity drugs.
- The natural aging process increases aromatase activity.
- Xenoestrogens – These are man-made chemicals that mimic estrogen in our bodies.
- Zinc deficiency.

Estrogen dominance will inhibit T4 to T3 conversion. Soy and fluoride do the same. Fluoride competes with iodine for absorption into your tissues and glands, including the thyroid. Fluoride has devastating effects on your enzymes. We need enzymes for all metabolic processes, including digestion and detoxification. Other side effects of fluoride include gastric distress, Down's syndrome, heart problems, headaches, breakdown of collagen protein, skin eruptions such as eczema and immune system problems.

Soy inhibits the thyroid gland. (See Chapter 2-4 for more on soy.) Healthy individuals without any previous thyroid disease were fed thirty grams of pickled soybeans per day for one month. (Ishizuki, et al.) Reports revealed goiter and elevated thyroid stimulating hormone (TSH) levels in thirty-seven healthy, iodine-sufficient adults. One month after stopping soybean consumption, individual TSH values decreased to the original levels and goiters were reduced in size.

People with an underactive fifth chakra tend to have thyroid issues. This may reveal itself as an individual who holds things in, such as emotions from a job they dislike or a relationship that lacks communication. When one is not honest with oneself, that person tends to have an underactive thyroid.

Focus on healing and restoring your adrenals. The health of your pancreas and your thyroid will usually return to functional operation when your adrenals are balanced.

The hormone you have the most control over is insulin. Insulin is managed by your diet and nutrition. Excess carbohydrates will raise your insulin levels. Consuming less than 1,800 calories per day will elevate insulin levels and decrease your brain chemistry. Control your insulin and you control your cortisol.

In order to stabilize your moods and avoid an increase in body fat, it is an important *Winning Formula* to eat every three to four hours.

If your liver is damaged and inflamed from the use of alcohol, prescription and/or OTC drugs or poor nutrition, you'll most likely have a weak response to any sort of hormone treatment, including Bio-Identical hormones.

Your liver has over 500 bodily functions. It is your body's filter system and lifeline. This organ produces cholesterol, lipoproteins and phospholipids. Your liver's detoxifying process depends on protein as it converts amino acids (proteins) and fats into glucose. The health of your body is dependent upon a healthy functioning liver. Your liver metabolizes hormone excesses and toxins, as well as fats and proteins. Increased protein intake in your diet encourages the breakdown of xenobiotics. Xenobiotics are chemicals or man-made substances not found in nature. Drugs such as antibiotics are a common xenobiotic.

Your liver assists in regulating your blood sugar levels. Your liver is affected by excessive consumption of alcohol.

Excessive consumption of alcohol is classified as two or more drinks per day. It takes your liver eight hours to detoxify one alcoholic beverage. Aside from liver damage and disease, excessive alcohol is high in empty calories with zero nutritional value. Excessive consumption contributes to significant health problems such as reactive hypoglycemia, obesity, hypertension as well as vitamin and mineral deficiencies.

Protect your liver. Certain foods, herbs and supplements can help detoxify, strengthen and improve liver function. Choline, found in cauliflower and cabbage, milk thistle, goldenseal, dandelion root tea, alpha lipoic acid and fresh lemon juice with water are nourishing *Winning Formulas* for your liver. Coconut oil helps your liver by keeping the bile ducts open. Deep breathing, castor oil packs, brisk daily walking, mini trampoline and regular saunas are other ways to maintain the health of your liver. It is also important to drink enough water.

Without a healthy liver, your body is destined for sub-performance and early death. An individual will have difficulty losing body fat if their liver is overburdened and congested with toxins. A healthy liver is critical for athletic performance, mental acuity, hormonal balance and skin health.

Symptoms of a toxic, congested liver include:

- Candida overgrowth
- Cellulite on a thin body
- Consistently waking up between the hours of 1:00 a.m. to 3:00 a.m.
- Constipation
- Depression
- Distended abdomen (men who are thin everywhere else, but stomach protrudes)
- Elevated cholesterol
- Food and chemical sensitivities
- Frequent illnesses
- Gallstones
- Gas or discomfort that is worse after a fatty meal
- Intolerance of smoke, perfume, or chemical fumes such as diesel
- Kidney disease
- Metallic taste in the mouth (this may also be a gallbladder issue or heavy metal toxicity)
- Pain in between the shoulder blades
- PMS
- Poor digestion

- Skin conditions (eczema, psoriasis, acne, rosacea, age spots)
- Tenderness with pressure applied at the middle of the front of the third rib
- Unexplained fatigue and headaches
- Unexplained weight gain
- Unresolved and repressed anger
- Unusually high cholesterol levels
- Weird dreams
- Yellow or white tongue

Suggested *Winning Formula* lab testing:

Fasting test. Always ask for a copy of your results.

- Adrenal Stress Index (saliva): 4 rhythm cortisol
- Candida (optional)
- CBC with differential
- CDSA – Comprehensive Digestive Stool Analysis (optional)
- C-Reactive Protein
- Homocysteine
- IGF-1 (optional)
- Iodine
- RBC magnesium or serum magnesium
- Serum glucose and insulin
- Serum iron and ferritin
- SMAC 25 to include GGTP (GGT)
- Thyroid panel: T3 (total, free or uptake), T4 (total or free, free thyroxine index and TSH (Serum or saliva testing)
- Total cholesterol, HDL, LDL, triglycerides
- Vitamin D, 25- Hydroxycalciferol

Suggested *Winning Formula* lab testing for females:
• Female Hormone Profile: Pregnenolone, Total Estrogens, DHEA-S, Progesterone, Testosterone (total) • N-Telopeptide, Urine

Suggested *Winning Formula* lab testing for males:
• Male Hormone Profile: Pregnenolone, Total Estrogens, DHEA, Progesterone, Bioavailable Testosterone, Testosterone (total), Testosterone (free) • PSA (Test at age 50 for Caucasian; age 40 for African American)

BioIdentical Hormones: In Europe, bioidentical hormones have been used by women for decades. Bioidenticals are plant-derived molecularly identical replicas of the hormones naturally produced by the human body. Prescriptions for bioidentical hormones can be tailored to the specific needs of each individual, allowing for flexibility in administration and dosage. It is best done with the help of a physician who specializes in anti-aging medicine or hormonal balance. Numerous studies published in highly respected international journals have demonstrated the safety and efficacy of bio-identical hormone replacement therapy.

150

CHAPTER 3-5

THE POWER OF LIFESTYLE

VALUE SYSTEM

"What is morality or ethics? A code of values to guide our choices and actions that decide, direct and develop the purpose and course of our lives."
~Ayn Rand

A unique characteristic of each individual is their value system. Realizing your own values and priorities are **Winning Formulas** for your personal growth, successful relationships and overall well-being.

A value can be viewed as a situation, entity or condition that you consistently make every effort to obtain, intend or preserve.

Many people talk about their beliefs, however very few have actually thought about their own value systems. Values are what drive your purpose for life. Your values strengthen and your appreciation of them escalates with consistent awareness and commitment of your time and energy.

Reassess and acknowledge what matters most to you. Decide what is essentially meaningful to you. This defines your quality of life.

Prioritize what is relevant and significant in the larger scheme of life. This can be thought-provoking and quite healing. This involves taking a look at how spiritually congruent you are – meaning how well you live your life with ethical and moral standards, integrity, authenticity and principles.

Evaluating your own personal value system opens the door to transformation to experience the gift of joy, inner peace and personal fulfillment. The outcome leads you directly to your destiny.

Winning Formulas to assess what your values are:

- A wide variety of options to decide upon.
- Choosing freely without input from your spouse, friends or relatives.
- Considering your options thoroughly.
- Committing to carrying out this value every day.

List your values in order of precedence and importance. Your personal *Winning Formula* value system may look something like this:

#1 – God

#2 – Self

#3 – Health

#4 – Friends, family, pets

#5 – Helping, empowering and inspiring others

#6 – Nature and the environment

#7 – Solitude, quiet and meditation

#8 – Work

Rank yourself high on your value list after God. This is not a selfish act. Realize that you are valuable. You are a priority. Otherwise, you are not able to be your best self for anyone or anything. Setting appropriate boundaries is a monumental *Winning Formula* in taking care of yourself. Give yourself permission to live a life influenced by your own personal value system. Living a life with balance is an essential *Winning Formula for Health, Vitality, Longevity and Fat Foss.* A balanced life leads to overall well-being on all levels – physically, emotionally, psychologically, intellectually and spiritually.

CHAPTER 3-6

WINNING FORMULAS FOR LIFESTYLE

"Love yourself! Do it now! Don't wait until you get well or lose the weight, or get the new job or the new relationship. Begin now – and do the best you can."
~Louise L. Hay

Choose two *Winning Formulas for Lifestyle* from the list below. Write your two *Winning Formulas* down on a piece of paper or post-it sticky note. Place them where they will be visible to you. Make copies. Keep them in several locations where you will see them easily.

- Apply a heating pad (not electric) on tense, tight muscles.
- Avoid aluminum cookware.
- Avoid xenoestrogens and estrogen precursors.
- Be aware and informed on the factors that create hormonal imbalances.
- Be aware of your thoughts. Switch from thoughts of deprivation to thoughts of abundance.
- Brush your teeth with fluoride-free toothpaste.
- Carve out at least five minutes daily to be quiet and still.
- Challenge your brain with mentally stimulating activities.

- Choose kind, healing words over gossip.
- Consciously be aware of your breathing patterns.
- Consciously reward yourself with stress-reducing activities or actions.
- Create an environment to promote a restful night's sleep around 8:00 p.m.
- De-clutter your home.
- Develop a practice of introspection.
- Dry brush your skin in an upward motion toward the heart before your shower or sauna to release toxins.
- Eliminate processed soy products from your diet.
- Encourage someone with a kind word, simple note or infectious smile.
- Find a like-minded support group.
- Forgive those who have broken your heart or angered you.
- Go to bed thirty minutes earlier every week until you are going to bed every night at 10:00 p.m.
- Have your mercury amalgams removed by a qualified dentist.
- If planning to become pregnant, both individuals should test for heavy metal toxicity.
- If you take synthetic thyroid medication, consult with a holistic, naturopathic medical practitioner for healthier alternatives.

- If approaching menopause, ask your doctor to test N-Telopeptide via urine analysis for bone density.

- Investigate possible causes of sleep disturbances.

- Journal your thoughts.

- Keep an open mind.

- Listen to soothing music.

- Log five things in your "Gratitude Journal" at the end of each day.

- Meditate and pray daily.

- Make a written list of your goals and update every three months.

- Practice diaphragmatic breathing at all stop lights.

- Recognize stress, sit in it and address it.

- Reduce exposure to environmental toxins – use water and air filters; natural personal care and cosmetics products, and biodegradable cleaning products.

- Refrain from judgment.

- Remove electromagnetic stressors from your bedroom.

- Schedule a monthly massage for yourself.

- Schedule an appointment for a thorough blood chemistry panel. (See pages 149 and 150.)

- Stay connected to those who are positive; disconnect from negative, toxic, energy vampires.

- Surround yourself with people who make you feel good.
- Test hormones via serum/blood testing.
- Test your thyroid at home with AM temperature readings.
- Trust your instincts; listen to your body.
- Tune out things that bring you down.
- Use natural cleaning products void of parabens and synthetic chemicals.
- Use natural personal care products void of parabens and synthetic chemicals.
- Volunteer or help those in need or who are less fortunate than you are.
- Wake up at the same time daily, approximately 6:00 a.m.
- Walk your dog or offer to walk your neighbor's dog (especially if the person is elderly and cannot walk his or her own dog).
- Watch a comedy.
- Work toward releasing any self-defeating thoughts of blame, self-pity or anger.
- Write down ten things that are most valuable to you in life.

See pages 100-102 for *Winning Formulas* for Sleep.

See pages 113-114 for *Winning Formulas* on Stress.

See pages 121-122 for *Winning Formula* Affirmations.

CHAPTER 4

THE POWER OF PHYSICAL EXERCISE

"Treat yourself and others with kindness when you eat, exercise, play, work, love and everything else."
~Dr. Wayne Dyer

Exercise is an essential *Winning Formula for Health, Vitality, Longevity and Fat Loss.* Exercise works regardless of age, race, and ethnic and genetic background. Moderate exercise is fundamental for a healthy functioning metabolism. There are some of you who exercise excessively. Others are completely sedentary. We sit and eat more, but move less. There are people who do way too much, too often. They wonder why their physiques remain unchanged. These are the individuals that always seem to be pushing it full throttle. With these individuals, less is more.

Excessive exercise leads to the degenerative diseases of aging. You're over-exercising if you exercise without eating enough food to support your activity level or if you do too much cardio day after day. Signs of over-exercising are painful joints or muscles several days after exercising, decreased range of motion, muscle breakdown, stiffness and swelling, injuries, hormonal imbalances and suppressed immune function.

Exercise bulimia is a disorder in which the individual's health is negatively affected physically, hormonally and psychologically from excessive amounts of exercise. Exercise bulimia is often connected to feelings of guilt about eating, and exercise is used as a form of purging. There is a deep-rooted emotional component attached with exercise bulimia as well as muscle dysmorphia, a disorder in which a person becomes obsessed that they are not muscular enough.

Excessive exercise increases free-radical oxidization. As mentioned earlier, we are hard-wired. Your physical body is not separate from your nervous, immune and endocrine systems. Your body does not distinguish stress from over-exercising to stress from an argument with your boss. When you exercise your immune system improves its functional capacity – yet, if you over-exercise it taxes your immune system, suppressing it.

If an individual is exercising sensibly and eating in a healthy way and still cannot lose weight, factors such as a damaged metabolism, emotional issues, adrenal burnout and insulin resistance should be considered. A damaged metabolism occurs from living with chronic states of stress, insufficient sleep, excessive use of stimulants and/or prescription medication, inadequate caloric intake and dieting, poor nutrition and over- or under-exercising. You can heal your metabolism implementing the principles of *THE POWER OF 4.*

Benefits of moderate exercise:

- Diffuses negative emotions such as anger, anxiety and depression
- Encourages other positive lifestyle changes
- Enhances cognitive and brain function
- Enhances your ability to deal with stress
- Improves posture
- Improves your overall sense of well-being
- Increased HDL cholesterol
- Increases energy
- Increases oxygen to tissues
- Increases self-esteem and self-confidence
- Increases serotonin production naturally without the use and side effects of antidepressants
- Prevents fatty liver disease
- Prevents osteoporosis by increasing bone mineral density
- Reduces structural stress
- Sheds unwanted body fat
- Stabilizes moods

Olympic Strength Coach, Charles Poliquin, has done extensive research on body composition. He developed BioSignature Modulation which is a twelve-site body fat caliper test that correlates where you deposit your body fat to how your hormonal system is functioning.

Genetically, we all have a pre-set number of fat cells at birth. The amount of body fat at each site relates to the levels of certain hormones in your body.

For instance, storing excess fat around your belly button indicates a long term exposure to cortisol. Your adrenals (stress glands) would need to be addressed. Excess body fat at the naval also indicates a need to reduce stimulants, manage stress, sleep more and eliminate simple sugars.

Insulin, secreted from your pancreas, is the hormone you have the greatest control over. It's the master hormone, as it influences all other hormones. Insulin is managed and controlled by regulating what you eat.

Fat around the iliac crest (hip bones) is a giveaway that you have been eating too many carbohydrates (sweets and junk food). Excess fat stored at the pectoral (chest) area or excess fat at the triceps site indicates testosterone imbalance. (See Chapter 3-4 for more on hormones.)

Stressors suppress androgens. (See Chapter 3-2 for more on lifestyle and stress.)

Stress can present in various forms such as:

- Emotional (divorce, financial problems, etc.)
- Environmental (pollution, electromagnetic, etc.)
- Physical (digestive issues, a sedentary lifestyle, marathon runners, etc.)

The area at the side of your ribs indicates thyroid imbalances. Excess body fat on your back, below the scapula, reveals that this individual displays a genetic inability to tolerating carbohydrates.

Your knees and calves are the growth hormone and pituitary sites. Excessive fat stores at the knee indicate a toxic, congested liver. The calf skin fold site is an indication of restful sleep and restoration. If you store fat in your knees or calves, you may not be sleeping well enough to secrete growth hormone. One of the many reasons to avoid anti-depressants is because they inhibit growth hormone causing you to gain weight. Growth hormone production occurs during sleep and when performing weight training exercise.

In females, excessive estrogen and too little progesterone is often the cause of excess body fat on the front and back of the thighs. (See page 142 for a list of natural estrogen inhibitors.)

After menopause or during times of extended stress, women tend to store more fat around their abdomens.

This often corresponds with a shift in hormone production. Before a woman experiences menopause, her adrenals produce forty percent of her sex hormones. After menopause her adrenals produce ninety percent of her sex hormones – more than her ovaries. During menopause and periods of stress, whether emotional, psychological or physical, this shows up as an "apple" shape in women.

According to researchers, "the higher a woman's percentage of body fat is at menopause, the more likely it is that she will suffer from night sweats and hot flashes."

We live in a 'quick fix society' where we want it now. People will do anything it takes to achieve what they want in the shortest amount of time with the least amount of effort, even if there are unhealthy consequences associated with it. Some people resort to liposuction. Charles Poliquin has found that liposuction causes the body to regain the amount of fat that has been surgically taken off and stores it in other places, especially around your organs, thus increasing risk of heart disease. Excessive internal body fat raises your risk of disease. Liposuction is not a natural process. Charles Poliquin has found that "when fat is removed by liposuction the body redistributes this fat on the upper arms, around the hips and at the side of the trunk (love handles or muffin top)."

To follow is my *Winning Formula* philosophy to empower you to create a leaner, healthier and stronger physique – naturally.

CHAPTER 4-1

THE POWER OF PHYSICAL EXERCISE

PERIODIZATION EQUALS PLANNING

"Every man is a builder of a temple called his body."
~Henry David Thoreau

Exercise and movement are ***Winning Formulas for Health, Vitality, Longevity and Fat Loss.*** Deciding to make a commitment to exercise is all part of your ***Winning Formula*** health equation. You are not meant to be sedentary. Choose something you enjoy doing. Commit to DO IT! There are endless activities at your disposal from which to choose.

Be determined and plan movement into your daily schedule. ***Winning Formula*** activities include: walking, gardening, strength training, biking, yoga, tai chi, hiking, swimming or Qi Gong.

If you've been sedentary for months or years, make a decision to start walking at a brisk pace every day, preferably outside. Start with twenty minutes daily. Progressively add ten more minutes each week until you're walking forty-five minutes at a time. Ask a friend to join you. This often helps with sticking to a routine. Brisk walking is great exercise because it's accessible, inexpensive, well-accepted among adults and has a low risk of injury.

You may wish to add hills and stairs as a ***Winning Formula*** for variety and as a way to add an interval element during your walks. Find a routine and be consistent with your physical exercise.

Your preference may be to exercise in the privacy of your home. There are several exercise DVDs available to select from. If your choice is weight training exercise at home, purchasing a stability ball and dumbbells can make for a perfect initial setup. Women would select dumbbells ranging in weight from five to thirty pounds. Men would select dumbbells up to fifty pounds. Strength training can also be done using your own bodyweight.

Daily bouncing on a mini trampoline stimulates circulation, gets your lymph moving and is highly beneficial for organ health. Your lymph serves as a pre-filter, screening out bacteria, viruses and debris to prevent clogging and overload on your liver. Your lymphatic system (lymph vessels and nodes, thymus gland, tonsils and spleen) produces white blood cells and antibodies, eliminates waste products from your tissues and carries your body's waste from your cells to your elimination organs.

Periodization sounds like a complex word. Quite simply, periodization is organized planning. Periodization is a variation of exercise programming. In regards to strength training, certain variables are systematically manipulated such as intensity, number of repetitions and sets, rest intervals, type of exercise, exercise tempo, type of contraction and frequency.

Your body has an incredible ability to adapt to any stress or demand placed upon it. The goal of periodization is to provide progressive and methodical overload, variety and specificity.

A 2002 study published in the Journal of Strength and Conditioning Research compared two different types of periodization – traditional linear periodization and undulating periodization. Traditional peridozation may work as follows: in weeks one through four you'd do eight reps per set of all your exercises. Weeks five through eight you'd do six reps. Weeks nine through twelve you'd do four reps.

Undulating periodization aims to achieve goals progressing from a hypertrophy protocol to one that emphasizes pure strength simultaneously. Undulating involves mixing or changing the training variables. Your week of training may look something like this: on Monday you'd do four reps per set, on Wednesday you'd do six reps and on Friday you'd do eight reps.

The researchers found that undulating periodization was far superior to linear periodization for strength gains and results.

Hire a qualified, professional fitness trainer. Have them design a resistance and stretching program specific to your goals and your lifestyle. Designing your own exercise program is like deciding to represent yourself in court.

Factors often overlooked in exercise programming are pattern overload, postural deviations, muscular imbalances and individual lifestyle. Your *Winning Formula* exercise program should correct postural imbalances, be matched to you specifically, balance out any muscular weaknesses, be specifically designed to your body type, increase your metabolism and factor in your overall lifestyle habits. Your exercise program should be moderately strenuous.

Posture can be enhanced with free weight training and functional exercise when working with a qualified practitioner. At the other end of the spectrum, your posture can deteriorate quickly when weight is added to your body per the direction of an unskilled practitioner causing further imbalances. Slumping from poor posture constricts your internal organs. Poor posture interferes with respiration, circulation and digestion. *Winning Formula* – Simply standing up straight gives you the appearance of looking five pounds thinner. Pull your shoulders back over your hips. Create length between the bottom of your rib cage and hips.

A qualified fitness expert will ensure your program is designed specific to you. In order to determine who is actually qualified as an expert, ask for references from friends who have had success.

168

The perpetual stereotype of a fitness trainer having a weak knowledge base, wearing inappropriate clothing, shouting orders and behaving unprofessionally still exists.

Winning Formulas of a professional fitness expert:

- A referral relationship with other medical and health professionals such as: Alternative Doctors, Nutritionists, Chiropractors, Orthopedic Physicians, Massage Therapists, Athletic Trainers, Occupational and Physical Therapists and other Personal Trainers.
- Act and look professional at all times; responsible; dependable.
- An educator that develops independence and empowers their clients.
- Certification and membership in professional organizations such as a Poliquin Performance Coach, CHEK, NASM, NSCA and ACSM.
- Certified in CPR (Cardio Pulmonary Resuscitation) and/or First Aid.
- Compatibility between you and the trainer.
- Consistent learning and stays on top of current trends and developments by attending seminars, conferences and continuing education.

- Excellent people skills and ability to communicate effectively.
- Great motivators who understand the process of change.
- Has the sense of when to refer out to other medical professionals when clients require services that are not within the trainer's "scope of practice." This basically means that the trainer should not provide advice that they are not trained to give.
- Help people achieve the results that they expect.
- If you are training for a specific reason, such as improved sports performance, the trainer should have relevant education and experience.
- Initially perform a full assessment of tests including movement screens, muscular length and tension, flexibility, body fat composition, girth measurements, postural analysis, as well as before and after photographs. The trainer should periodically re-test to monitor progress.
- Knowledge of exercise technique and exercise theory.
- Knowledge of human physiology and nutrition.
- Loyal and a high level of integrity.
- Passionate.
- Present themselves as a role model in mind, body and action. (Are they congruent?)
- Provide references.

CHAPTER 4-2

THE POWER OF PHYSICAL EXERCISE

RESISTANCE AND WEIGHT TRAINING

"Subjects in their mid-80s can return to a muscular biological age of someone in their mid-50s with only three months of strength training."
~Charles Poliquin

When it comes to **Health, Vitality, Longevity and Fat Loss**, weight training is the secret **Winning Formula** for anyone in search of the fountain of youth.

It's essential to overload your muscle tissue with weight or resistance exercise versus aerobic exercise, which breaks your body down. Increased muscle tissue protects your tendons, ligaments and joints. Leg and core strength have a significant, positive impact on your posture. Consistent resistance training has been shown to increase insulin sensitivity. This means your body can take in and use glucose more effectively, delivering glucose to your working muscles for energy production.

Resistance training works regardless of the person's conditioning level. Resistance training is far superior to aerobic exercise for altering body composition and prevention of obesity.

Resistance exercise promotes *Health, Vitality, Longevity and Fat Loss* making it the ultimate anti-aging *Winning Formula* activity. Causes of muscle aging include oxidative stress, cell death, inflammation, hormonal dysregulation, alterations in protein turnover, inactivity, and mitochondrial dysfunction.

Resistance weight training is associated with hypertrophy (gains in lean muscle mass). It may actually prevent and reverse bone loss! Researchers at Tufts University in Boston evaluated twelve biological markers that could predict longevity in individuals. To the amazement of the scientific community, the top two of these parameters turned out to be "muscle mass and level of strength."

Resistance training works to build muscle by forcing your body to heal the damage to your muscle cells that has occurred with use. When the intensity is high enough, microscopic tears occur in your muscle. It is after your resistance workout that muscle synthesis (rebuilding) occurs, resulting in hypertrophy and stronger muscles.

It is now known that previous studies done on older individuals lifting weights did not show a positive response because the participants were not using the correct exercise intensity, meaning the subjects were lifting weights that were too light.

The amount of muscle mass you have influences your ability to tolerate disease. Your body burns muscle and protein at a faster rate than usual when you're stressed or sick.

This causes protein to be pulled from your muscle tissue for your immune system to help fight the disease, stressor or illness.

One of the primary conditions of aging is "sarcopenia." This is the loss of neurons in the nervous system causing atrophy, a loss of muscle size, and decreased strength accompanied by an increase in fat storage under the skin. Sarcopenia occurs primarily in fast twitch muscle fibers. These muscle fibers are larger. They have faster contraction and firing action. Sarcopenia is a serious degenerative condition that increases your risk of accidental falls. Sarcopenia makes you more vulnerable to injury.

Researchers at Ball State University found that "strength training increased an individual's fast-twitch muscle fibers." These are the exact muscle fibers that diminish as you age. Fast-twitch muscle fibers produce greater muscle force than slow-twitch muscle fibers. Long, slow distance (LSD) aerobic exercise is a slow-twitch dominant exercise.

The good news is that sarcopenia is reversible by adhering to a sensible strength training program performed on a consistent basis.

If you want an exercise program that produces results faster, with the least amount of time put into it, resistance training is the *Winning Formula* exercise. Thirty to forty minutes of strength training, performed three times per week is adequate given that the exercise selection provides progressive overload, intensity and adequate stimuli to your muscular and nervous systems.

Muscle is your metabolically-active, fat burning tissue! For every additional pound of muscle on your physique, you burn an additional fifty calories per day, whereas each pound of fat burns a trivial two calories daily. Muscle tissue improves insulin resistance. Resistance training is highly beneficial for diabetics as it increases the number and the sensitivity of insulin receptors. Extra glucose goes to the muscle tissue, not the fat cells.

Your muscles require calories to survive and they like weight lifting. The more muscle you have, the more effectively you burn fat – providing you are not overly stressed.

One of the most prevalent mistakes routinely made by women in gyms all over the world – they don't lift heavy enough weights. In addition, they perform a high number of repetitions. One of the main complaints I often hear from females in their twenties, thirties, forties and up is that their legs are either fat or thick.

Upon observation, these women tend to spend a vast amount of time on cardiovascular exercise. Never or seldom do these women spend any time weight training. The bigger the woman, the lighter the weights she uses. She is afraid that lifting heavy dumbbells will make her even bigger. Observe the lean, tight and toned women. More often than not these women lift heavier weights.

The *Winning Formula* training program for estrogen-dominant legs is one which builds muscle. Proper nutrition must always be factored in.

Workouts involving the major muscles will force your body to lose the fat reserves and increase muscle mass. My *Winning Formula* exercises for lean, strong legs include: squats, multi-directional lunges, dead lifts and step ups.

Moderately- to highly-trained females are very capable of doing advanced multiple-set and multiple-exercise program designs as compared to males. Females are also able to complete frequent resistance training workouts on a weekly basis as compared to males because females have unique physiological and metabolic characteristics that make this possible.

Here is my analogy of fat versus muscle and the amount of space these tissues take up in your body. Muscle equals one pound of nuts and bolts (dense and takes up a small space). Fat equals one pound of cotton balls (occupies much space).

Muscle mass can increase without your legs appearing bigger because the composition changes. The amount of intramuscular fat diminishes with strength training. Using light weights and a high number of repetitions will not achieve this effect. The only time lighter weights and higher repetitions are recommended is during the intro phase for trainees who do not have experience and need to strengthen their joints and tendons first. This initial phase helps create quality motor engrams of various exercises. Exercise technique and quality of movement are *Winning Formulas* for injury prevention and results.

Ideally, weight training routines should be periodized (planned variation and manipulation) every four to six weeks for consistent change and progression. The older you are in 'training years,' the more often you benefit from a change in program design. This also ensures prevention from boredom. Periodization avoids complacency, pattern overload and neurological adaptation.

Resistance exercise has been shown to have a dramatic effect on hormonal responses in your body after exercise training. A May 2007 study from the *Public Library of Science* revealed the "dramatic potential for resistance training to reverse the aging effect of muscle." All hormones in your body have an influence on the aging process. Hormones are affected by weight training. Growth hormone, IGF-1 and testosterone released from resistance exercise have an effect on muscle hypertrophy, increased bone mass and enhanced quality skin texture.

Resistance training programs should be designed to increase muscular strength, power and hormonal response. The program should correct postural imbalances and muscular weaknesses. Training to failure is not recommended. This will actually make individuals more susceptible to injury and overtraining. Overtraining affects hormone production and muscular power adaptations, thus increasing inflammation. It creates a sympathetic dominant nervous system. Two common triggers of overtraining in resistance training are excessive volume and excessive intensity.

In a unique study (Izquierdo, et al, 2006); hormonal responses of resistance training to failure versus not-to-failure were examined. The study revealed that the "not-to-failure group showed greater increases in strength and power. Also, increases in insulin-like growth factor 1 (IGF-1) and resting testosterone levels, as well as greater reductions in cortisol."

Your body tends to acclimate quickly to the demands placed upon it. The number one approach to vary a weight training routine is created by manipulating repetitions and sets. Never spend more than four weeks in one repetition zone. Other variables that influence your resistance training exercise program design include the exercise selection, order of exercises performed, rest interval length and tempo of the exercise.

Alwyn Cosgrove says, "If you want to become stronger, stay away from weight machines. They are a sure method for becoming overall weaker, less efficient and more injury prone. Lift either your body weight or a free weight such as a barbell, dumbbell, kettlebell or sandbag through space. Always use exercises that make you move more than one joint at a time. Isolation exercises like biceps curls are only useful for body builders. To make your time more efficient, you can superset upper and lower body exercises such as a deadlift alternated with a push press, and repeat for sets so that you workout is compressed."

Strength training doesn't necessarily require weights. California banned weightlifting in their prisons and found out that the inmates become faster, stronger, more flexible and more dangerous as they switched from lifting weights to training only with their body weight. These concepts should give you some ideas on how to exercise in less time, at less cost and with more results.

Around forty years of age loss of muscle and deficits in strength begin to occur. Strength training becomes more important as we age. Generally, I recommend strength training a minimum of two days per week and up to four days weekly for approximately forty-five minutes each session. *Winning Formula* exercises are multi-joint, big bang exercises. These include dead lifts, push ups, lunges, step ups, pull ups, squats, push presses and various compound movements. Keep your sets to no more than sixty seconds in length and rest for at least sixty seconds between sets.

The amount of muscle mass you have also indicates how healthy you are, how well you will age and the effectiveness of your immune system. Weight training is a drug-free, anti-aging *Winning Formula* antidote.

When you restrict your calories by dieting, or if excessive cortisol is causing your muscles to atrophy, your metabolic rate will slow down. This causes fewer calories to be burned during your everyday activities. These excess calories will be stored as fat. This is an ideal environment to increase body fat!

When the speed of your metabolism is increased, your muscle cells want more energy from your fat stores. They use more fat per hour compared to when your metabolism is slower or temporarily revved up. Weight training elevates your metabolism for one to two days afterwards.

In conjunction with weight training, eating an adequate amount of protein will encourage muscle hypertrophy. You will feel stronger and accelerate your fat burning furnace.

Winning Formula – as you lose unwanted body fat toxins diminish from within your body. Toxins accumulate in your fat tissue.

Upon completion of your weight training workout, post-exercise nutrition is critical, ideally within thirty minutes afterwards. A high-quality whey protein isolate is a beneficial ***Winning Formula*** to include after exercise. Whey protein is one of the most quickly absorbed types of protein. Good carbohydrate sources post-workout include bananas or honey. Whey protein ingestion stimulates protein synthesis by sixty-eight percent, while casein protein ingestion stimulates protein synthesis at only thirty-one percent. In addition, amino acids, glutamine, arginine and leucine, have important roles in muscle protein metabolism. Casein protein contains 11.6 and 8.9 grams of these amino acids, respectively while whey protein contains 21.9 and 11.1 grams of these amino acids, respectively.

Thus, the enhanced digestion rate of the whey protein may be more important than the amino acid composition of the protein. (See Chapter 2-5 for more on whey protein.)

An Arizona State University study revealed benefits of whey protein on muscle protein anabolism are due to something other than its amino acid content. The authors conclude, "This finding may have practical implications for the formulation of nutritional supplements to enhance muscle anabolism in older individuals."

Exercise causes oxidative damage and breakdown of tissue. Post-exercise nutrition decreases cortisol and increases growth hormone. Post-work out nutrition repairs your muscle tissue creating protein and muscle synthesis plus replenishing muscle glycogen.

A recent study confirmed that "due to the high levels of polyphenols, mainly catechins, consumption of green tea may offer protection against the oxidative damage caused by exercise." The potential protective health effects from the catechins have been attributed to antioxidant, anti-thrombogenic and anti-inflammatory properties. Green tea is rich in antioxidants and may protect the body by raising the level of glutathione, a protein that helps prevent oxidative damage.

Drinking green tea is a *Winning Formula* for health, vitality, longevity and fat loss, and has many life-extending benefits.

180

Green tea catechins combined with exercise helps decrease abdominal fat and triglycerides in overweight adults.

Individuals with abdominal obesity are three times more likely to develop dementia and sixty-three percent more likely to develop cancer. (Zhang, C et al, 2008).

Green tea extract is a proficient estrogen blocker. Regular consumption of green tea is associated with a slightly lower risk of breast cancer, according to the Shanghai Breast Cancer Study.

Green tea extracts have a cholesterol lowering effect which can be used to prevent the absorption of cholesterol from the intestinal tract. Green tea appears to stimulate the biliary elimination of cholesterol from the liver.

In addition, drinking green tea is very effective in temporarily reducing halitosis because of its disinfectant and deodorant activities. Green tea may help alleviate sleep-disordered breathing such as obstructive sleep apnea.

Remember, green tea does contain caffeine and is best to consume the caffeinated variety earlier in the day.

Benefits of resistance strength training:

- Decreases both total and intra-abdominal fat
- Diminishes low back pain
- Effective intervention against sarcopenia
- Elevates resting metabolism
- Healthier digestion
- Improves cholesterol levels
- Improves function and reduces pain in those with osteoarthritis in the knee region
- Lessens stress
- Muscle hypertrophy (growth)
- Normalizes blood pressure in those with high normal values
- Prevents the loss of BMD (bone mineral density)
- Produces substantial increases in strength, mass, power and quality of skeletal muscle
- Reduces insulin resistance as well as enhances glucose metabolism
- Reduces risk factor for falls
- Stronger connective tissue

CHAPTER 4-3

THE POWER OF PHYSICAL EXERCISE

DE-STRESS AND FLEXIBILITY

"The greater the difficulty, the more glory in surmounting it."
~Epicurus

Stretching and de-stressing exercises are powerful *Winning Formulas* to relieve tension and tight muscles. As you age, it is very important that you remain supple. We lose elasticity in our muscles and tendons as we age. Excessive tension in your muscles and organs rob you of vital energy.

Some of you are inflexible and stiff. You have many muscle groups that are overly contracted and tight. This scenario requires an increase in flexibility. If your body is in a constant state of contraction, you risk pulling a muscle from excessive tension. Your focus should be on increasing flexibility, joint mobilization and optimal tissue length.

On the other hand, some of you have musculoskeletal systems that are too loose. You'd be considered "hypermobile." You have greater risk of injury from a trauma or an activity like running that creates a great amount of impact forces on your joints.

An individual who is hypermobile lacks the strength to stabilize his or her joints. They would benefit from a program of strengthening their connective and muscular tissue.

As you age, it takes longer to recover from the stress of a hard workout. Build in more rest days, allow for recover and stretch daily.

Benefits of stretching:

- Better posture
- Eliminate or reduce low back pain
- Feels good
- Greater circulation
- Improve joint range of motion
- Increase flexibility
- Reduce muscle and fascia tightness
- Reduce physiological stress

Static stretching is the type of stretching most people are familiar with. In reality, there are a variety of stretching techniques.

Types of stretching:

Active Isolated Stretching (AIS): AIS consists of assuming a position, then holding it there for two seconds which allows the target muscle to lengthen without triggering the stretch reflex. The theory is that as one muscle contracts, the opposing muscle relaxes, known as reciprocal inhibition, which increases motor-neuron excitability allowing muscles to elongate. AIS is an effective, dynamic and facilitated type of stretching technique.

Ballistic Stretching: Ballistic stretching consists of trying to force a part of your body beyond its normal range of motion by bouncing into a stretched position. An example of ballistic stretching would be bouncing down repeatedly to touch your toes. Although ballistic stretching does have its place, it can lead to injury and is best utilized by those who need to prepare for high-speed activity.

Dynamic Stretching: Dynamic stretching is performed with continuous, controlled movement using active muscular effort to increase your range of motion gradually without holding the end position. Dynamic stretching prepares your body for the imposed demands that are to be placed upon it. It stimulates the nervous system. Dynamic stretching is an ideal warm up prior to an exercise program.

Fascial Stretch Therapy™: *Stretch to Win* founder, Ann Frederick, created Fascial Stretch Therapy™ which focuses on stretching and aligning your fascia. Fascia is your connective tissue – the most influential structure in your body affecting your flexibility. Age, trauma, injuries, poor posture and inadequate training can distort, twist and tighten the fascia. Changes to the fascia can cause major and minor imbalances in strength, speed, flexibility, balance and agility, but usually the cause goes undetected because most individuals do not stretch the fascia.

Isometric Stretching: Isometric stretching consists of getting a muscle into a stretched position and then resisting the stretch isometrically. An example of isometric stretching would be standing in a doorway with hands up to ear level on the doorjambs, applying force against the doorway to open up the chest muscles.

Static Stretching: Static stretching is the most common type of stretching. Static stretching is a form of stretching where the actual stretch is held for thirty to ninety seconds. There is no movement with static stretching. You may feel slight discomfort as the muscles and connective tissues lengthen. This type of stretching is best performed at the end of a workout or before bedtime. It is calming and provides a parasympathetic response to your nervous system.

Proprioceptive Neuromuscular Facilitation (PNF): PNF is a technique combining passive and isometric stretching together to achieve maximum flexibility. PNF was originally developed by physical therapists for rehabilitation purposes. PNF consists of a muscle being passively stretched, then contracted isometrically against resistance while in the stretched position and passively stretched again through the resulting increased range of motion. PNF is usually performed with the assistance of a partner who provides resistance against the isometric contraction and then takes the muscle through its increased range of motion.

Exercises such as yoga, Tai Chi, meditative walks and Qi Gong provide internal energy. They produce fresh energy in your body. The combination of movement and deep, full breathing techniques allow tension and stress to dissipate from your body.

Inadequate or shallow breathing patterns create tension in your physical body. Something as simple as deep, full belly breathing from your diaphragm is very healing and nourishing physiologically. Deep breathing creates internal physiological transformation at a cellular level.

Yoga, Qi Gong, Tai Chi and stretching release physical and emotional tension. They provide you with extra energy to deal with everyday life creating feelings of calm, serenity and inner peace.

Tai Chi and Qi Gong are Chinese martial arts that involve slow, fluid movement, breathing and meditation. Thousands of Asian studies confirm Qi Gong as a great harmonizer of body and mind with remarkable healing properties. In an article published in the American Journal of Public Health researchers found that Tai Chi showed improvements in overall functional independence (being able to perform daily tasks without help) and improved balance.

Consistent yoga practice creates a healing power outside of the actual practice itself in which transformation of the mind takes place. Yoga is a powerful, natural therapy for many diseases and health conditions. Yoga can dramatically shift your unhealthy, unsupportive emotions into constructive and helpful ones, helping you to experience happy, content lives.

Yoga releases energetic blockages called *granthis* in Sanskrit. These are knots that form at the navel region, the seat of personal power; the heart center, the seat of the emotional body, and the throat, the seat of self-expression. When these blockages are released, your physical and emotional layers open and energy flows freely. This energy, called *prana*, is the essential life-force of all beings. When prana flows freely through your body, you feel vital and healthy; you reconnect with others and become a part of the world.

Benefits of yoga:

- Better posture
- Biochemical advantages
- Calms the central nervous system and stimulates the parasympathetic nervous system
- Connection with universal energy
- Decreases stress and tension
- Enhances balance and flexibility
- Improves symptoms of metabolic syndrome
- Improves certain symptoms of back pain
- Improves symptoms of carpal tunnel syndrome (if focus is on upper body)
- Internal awareness (breath)
- Non-competitive, process oriented
- Psychological advantages
- Reduces perceived severity and duration of hot flashes
- Releases energetic blockages
- Relieves common symptoms of osteoarthritis
- Stimulates digestion
- Sub-cortical region of the brain is stimulated
- Tones muscles and joints

According to a survey conducted at Royal Melbourne Institute of Technology University, "more people are participating in yoga for mental and emotional complaints, such as anxiety, fear, stress, depression and sleep disorders than for physical ailments." Ninety-six percent of the people who practiced yoga noticed improvements in their health. Women acknowledged relief from menstrual and menopausal symptoms.

Deepak Chopra quotes, *"Any reason for practicing yoga is a good reason. Enhancing flexibility and releasing stress are as noble a purpose for performing yoga as the awakening of spirituality. This is the great gift of yoga – it serves and nourishes us at every level of your being and spontaneously contributes to greater well-being in all domains of life. Yoga will help you discover gifts within yourself that have remained unopened since your childhood – gifts of peace, harmony, laughter and love."*

Pilates emphasizes precision and control. It teaches concentration, awareness of your breath and alignment of your spine. Pilates improves your mental and physical well-being, increases flexibility and coordination as well as strengthens deep-torso muscles.

De-stressing exercises produce feelings of relaxation and overall **Health, Vitality, Longevity** and contentment. Additional benefits establish a reduction in both, physiological and psychological stress, clearing out the mental toxins of the day.

CHAPTER 4-4

THE POWER OF PHYSICAL EXERCISE

REDUCE LSD

"Walking is man's best medicine."
~Hippocrates

LSD is an acronym for long, slow distance training, not a hallucinogenic drug!

In the late 1960s and early 1970s aerobic exercise was introduced to the masses by Dr. Kenneth Cooper, known as the "father of aerobics." Dr. Cooper's thirty years of research clearly revealed the benefits of aerobic exercise on the pulmonary and cardiovascular systems.

Walking two to three miles in thirty minutes, three days per week will reduce your risk of heart attack by almost sixty percent. Moderate- and fast-paced walking is a ***Winning Formula*** that will definitely elevate your HDL cholesterol. However, an hour or more of aerobics, normally in the form of LSD jogging, cycling, marathon training, spinning and boot camp classes has been proven to be an ineffective method of exercise for most sports. More importantly, damaging to your metabolism and unproductive for improving your body's ability to burn and lose body fat!

Continuous aerobic work plateaus after eight weeks of training. Anything more is really counterproductive. While it may be true that aerobic exercise may help you lose fat initially, it is not an efficient method for altering your body composition. If your life is stressful, adding more stress by doing too much continuous LSD aerobic work will actually increase your body fat.

Your body adapts to any stressor placed upon it. What used to take thirty minutes to burn three hundred calories will soon take forty minutes of your time, then, forty-five minutes, then, an hour and so on. You're creating the perfect environment to efficiently store body fat!

We've been brainwashed to believe that the more aerobic exercise we do, the better our hearts will function. We think we'll burn more body fat, live longer and look better. Nothing could be further from the truth.

Long, slow distance (LSD) aerobic exercise is very time-consuming when you weigh the benefits as compared to resistance training. Long, slow distance (LSD) exercise tends to accelerate the aging process. It creates inflammation in your body due to the excessive buildup of oxidative stress as a byproduct from aerobic training. LSD is time-consuming when evaluating the pros and cons. What's more, LSD is unnecessary. It can lead to insulin resistance and create additional imbalances, especially hormonally.

Research indicates that high-intensity (>70% of maximal effort) exercise sessions lasting longer than 20-30 minutes or low intensity (< 50%-70%) efforts lasting longer than 75 minutes can flood the body with stress and inflammation biochemical markers, initiating a cascading response (Borer 2003; Tiidus 2008).

Evidence suggests that when you exercise excessively your immune system is suppressed. This is evidenced in distance runners that show an elevated incidence of upper respiratory tract infections.

The problem with using aerobic exercise as a method for altering your body composition is two-fold: whether the intensity is too high or too low, either way you burn very little fat. Fat must be converted through a series of enzymes into a substance your body can use.

For an individual who is insulin-resistant, aerobic exercise is the worst exercise prescription for them. Aerobic exercise causes an insulin-resistant or diabetic person to become fatter. Weight training is the perfect *Winning Formula* exercise of choice for a diabetic. Resisted strength training enhances muscle growth (hypertrophy). The number and sensitivity of insulin receptors increase with resistance weight training exercise. This causes extra glucose to go into the muscle tissue versus the fat cells.

Your metabolism does not remain elevated with aerobic exercise. Aerobic exercise burns calories for the time spent doing the activity. You burn very few calories once you stop the exercise. However, your metabolism does remain elevated with resistance exercise. This increased energy used after an intelligent workout is referred to as excess post-exercise oxygen consumption (EPOC). EPOC is a physiological payment of oxygen debt. Aerobic exercise creates a minimal oxygen debt. EPOC is a measure of how much oxygen the body consumes in the hours and days after a workout.

One must exercise for long durations and often (at least five or more times per week) in order to burn any amount of fat with LSD. This is how long distance runners maintain their slim physiques. HOWEVER, when a runner sustains an injury and is unable to train their metabolism spirals down. This leads to increased body fat over time. This affects women more rapidly than men. The effects are magnified for women in their late thirties and early forties as a woman approaches menopause. The constant speeding up and slowing down of a woman's metabolism from years of LSD has adverse hormonal implications. Combine this with stress or an injury and she finds that aerobic exercise no longer keeps her slim. Most aerobic training is dependent on an emotional attachment to it.

Even if your sport of choice is purely endurance-based, such as marathon running, triathlon, long distance cycling or cross-country skiing, your exercise program should be designed accordingly for optimal performance gains and injury prevention.

This requires proper prescription of the exercise program variables to maximize the benefits associated with resistance and interval training. Proper program design is that which incorporates progressive overload, variation and specificity.

LSD training for sport or any other reason has been shown to "restrict mobility, increase your chances of repetitive strain injuries and break down muscle tissue in order to retain your body's natural homeostasis." LSD exercise decreases power. It creates a *slower* athlete.

The majority of sports require short bursts of effort interspersed with periods of rest known as interval training or anaerobic exercise. Think of a golf swing, one hundred meter sprint, darting across the basketball court, a tennis stroke or rushing at an opponent to make a tackle.

The ability of your body to handle these efforts is based on the ability of your muscles to recover efficiently and be prepared for the next effort.

An interval-based training plan has been shown to be NINE times more effective for fat loss than doing LSD workouts, such as jogging or working out on an exercise bike for an hour or more!

An interval-based program improves BOTH aerobic and anaerobic fitness. Interval training programs are short in duration. This means the total amount of actual work out time is usually no more than fifteen minutes. This is a "true" interval program.

Examples of interval training:

- Forty seconds of effort with two minutes active rest or ten seconds effort and sixty seconds active rest.

- Six seconds of all-out effort with nine seconds of rest.

- Allow your heart rate to elevate to 140 beats per minute (bpm) and keep it there for sixty seconds. Allow your heart rate to recover to ninety bpm or lower for approximately one to two minutes and repeat.

- The ultimate interval program is a total workout of eight to twelve minutes with intervals of thirty to sixty seconds of effort followed by thirty seconds of rest.

An interval workout that alternates resistance training with a high intensity sprint has one of the greatest effects on body composition. This style of training most closely represents the way athletes train, and is also the most likely type of training humans evolved with.

It's extremely important to eliminate LSD if you're suffering from adrenal fatigue. Any time your heart rate is 100 beats or higher cortisol is released and epinephrine is stimulated. Epinephrine usually breaks down fat for energy.

However, when both cortisol and epinephrine are elevated at the same time, fat cells become unresponsive to breaking down fat. Instead, metabolically-active lean muscle tissue is broken down. Obviously, this is not an ideal fat loss or anti-aging protocol.

Stopping high-intensity aerobic work is more important as you age. Your adrenal glands produce forty percent of your sex hormones before menopause and ninety percent after menopause.

Resistance exercise works regardless of your conditioning level. This type of training produces more "bang for your buck." Resistance exercise is the ultimate *Winning Formula* exercise for *Health, Vitality, Longevity and Fat Loss.*

World-renowned, Olympic strength coach, Charles Poliquin, voices his opinion on aerobic exercise. Charles' famous quote is: *"Don't do aerobic work; it makes you dumber and fatter."*

Charles Poliquin's opinion is in exact agreement with those of Paul Chek and Dr. Diana Schwarzbein, an endocrinologist who studies the hormonal effects of food and exercise. Dr. Schwarzbein says, *"Nobody needs cardio."*

LSD exercise is problematic because it causes cortisol to rise unopposed by the growth-promoting hormones, testosterone and growth hormone. This creates a physical stress response to your entire body. Prolonged release of cortisol, whether from long-term physical, mental or emotional stress, or the wrong kind of exercise, atrophies (shrinks) your muscles, nerves and brain cells.

This may explain why standard aerobic exercise is not effective for optimal body composition and why marathon runners exhibit frail bodies devoid of muscle. The duration – not the intensity – of the exercise is the most significant issue in regards to cortisol.

Chronic over-secretion of cortisol causes a weakened immune system, a decrease in lean muscle, hair loss, thinning skin, infertility, inability to grow nails and a decrease in concentration and memory. Excess cortisol kills brain cells, including those in the hippocampus, where the brain processes emotions. Excessive cortisol production can also deplete serotonin levels causing depression.

If you desire real transformation, want to combat obesity and ensure fat loss, you must exercise for metabolic acceleration to make this happen. Short-duration, high-intensity exercise versus LSD exercise is the *Winning Formula* exercise prescription.

Do you want to be a fat-storing machine or an accelerated fat loss machine? Plain and simple – STOP THE INSANE LSD TRAINING!

CHAPTER 4-5

THE POWER OF PHYSICAL EXERCISE

ACTIVE REST AND HEALING

"The secret of health for both mind and body is not to mourn for the past, not to worry about the future, or not to anticipate troubles, but to live the present moment wisely and earnestly."
~Buddha

Anything done in excess creates imbalances physically, emotionally and spiritually. This may include excessive exercise, over-working and/or substance abuse. Allowing time for restoration and relaxation each and every day is a definite *Winning Formula*. The end result is a state of balance and overall well-being on all levels.

There are various forms of healing that do not rely on pharmaceutical drugs or surgery. Alternative healing therapies are actually more cost-effective in the long run. They emphasize prevention. Alternative healing remedies deal with the cause, rather than the symptoms. They allow your body to heal itself. These healing remedies do not promote drugs which cause side effects and require yet another drug.

Winning Formula healing therapies:

- Acupuncture
- Applied Kinesiology (AK)
- Aromatherapy
- Bio-feedback
- Chiropractic care

- Color Therapy
- Emotional Freedom Technique (EFT)
- Hypnotherapy
- Massage
- Meditation

- Prayer
- Reflexology
- Reiki
- Rest from exercise
- Restorative Yoga
- Sound Therapy

Faith and spirituality have a powerful effect on health. **Prayer,** a powerful form of medicine, provides faith and hope. Prayer is the oldest and most popular form of spiritual self-care. The latest research shows that prayer can actually improve the growth rate of cell cultures, seeds, plants, fungi and bacteria. Prayer is a form of communication with God. My belief is that when we are still and quiet with ourselves our intuition is highly activated. This is when we can hear God speaking to us. There are over 200 recent studies revealing that spirituality and faith speed recovery from illness and surgery, boosts immune response and extends lifespan.

Acupuncture and acupressure are ancient systems of Traditional Chinese Medicine that encourage your body to heal naturally. The goal of acupuncture is to balance your vital energy by stimulating specific points along the body's meridians or energy channels. This is done by inserting needles and applying heat or other stimulation at these precise points. Acupuncture has been shown to be effective for acute and chronic health conditions.

Applied kinesiology (AK) is a Traditional Chinese Medicine technique which can determine health imbalances in your body's organs and glands by identifying weaknesses in specific muscles.

Applied kinesiology is based on the principle that muscles, glands and organs are all linked by meridians or energy pathways within the body. It works by restoring balanced energy flow.

Aromatherapy is the use of essential oils from natural plant essences and herbs to treat a range of health conditions. Aromatherapy acts on your central nervous system relieving depression and anxiety and reducing stress. Aromatherapy can be relaxing, uplifting, sedating or stimulating, thus restoring both physical and emotional well-being. Essential oils have been used throughout Europe for over 120 years.

Chiropractic adjustments are effective for relieving pain and improving structural well-being and overall health. These adjustments focus on maintaining and restoring health through aligning your musculoskeletal structure to improve your body's functions. Every nerve in the body passes through the spine. When not in alignment, your nervous system is affected creating pain and discomfort. Your spinal nerves are responsible for feeling pain and for movement of muscles. Slight distortions in your spine, muscle imbalances, poor posture and body mechanics, old injuries and tightness all create pain and stress on your body and its various organs. Chiropractic care provides healing and promotes good health by helping your nervous system to function optimally.

The rainbow, a healing key, contains a full spectrum of color and is a symbol of abundance, completion, potential and possibility. Each color is energy vibrating at a different frequency and wavelength.

Every color has its own attributes to which you are both consciously and subconsciously attuned. Various colors influence your body's chemistry and balance affecting you physically, emotionally, psychologically and spiritually. Color therapy is the use of color and light to balance the flow of energy throughout your body.

The **Emotional Freedom Technique (EFT)** is a simple, direct approach to release and redirect blocked energy patterns in the body and mind. Through a simple tapping technique core emotional issues, as well as physical difficulties, often clear quickly and easily. As with acupuncture and acupressure techniques, EFT works through releasing blocks in the flow of energy along meridian lines. This form of "emotional acupressure" follows a pattern of tapping on specific meridian points. Tapping while focusing your attention on a specific problem or area of concern stimulates the meridians to help release emotional blocks, rebalance the flow of energy, support emotional well-being and promote healing at a cellular level.

Hypnotherapy is a form of deep relaxation bringing calmness to the mind and access to the subconscious. In a state of hypnosis, you remain calm and aware of all that is said, the sounds and environment around you. You feel relaxed and engrossed in the moment.

The intent of hypnotherapy is to assist in re-programming a behavior or mindset to provide more meaningful alternatives to limiting thoughts, circumstances and patterns.

Massage therapy is the use of touch applied to heal your body, promote relaxation and reduce tension. Massage is effective for promoting the recovery process from exercise. Massage therapy provides a sedative effect on your nervous system, increases lymphatic circulation and helps break up scar tissue, to list a few.

Meditation is the integration of your mind and body with deep breathing and focused attention. The practice has been used for thousands of years. Meditation is one of the most natural *Winning Formula* techniques you can practice to increase your immunity quickly and effectively. It helps you feel more at peace, creating calm within, especially on an emotional level.

While meditation is usually thought to be done in a seated position, it can be done lying down, standing or during slow walking.

Meditation provides healing by opening up the paths of communication between your brain and body and by quieting your mind. In fact, meditation helps you sustain energy. Meditation is powerful, with over 500 scientific studies revealing numerous health benefits.

Reflexology is founded on a system of healing that works through stimulation of the feet. All organs, glands and structures of your body can be mapped from and accessed through your feet. This gentle form of massage applies pressure to specific parts of your feet in order to promote relaxation, detoxification, release and healing elsewhere in your body. The treatment can help restore balance and energy flow throughout your body. As with most healing modalities, reflexology works with your body's natural energy, or Qi (pronounced "Chi"), by stimulating internal pathways for energy (called "meridians") all of which are accessible through your feet.

Reiki is a Japanese technique used for stress reduction and relaxation that also promotes healing. It's based on the idea that an unseen "life force energy" flows through us and is what causes us to be alive. If your "life force energy" is low, you are more likely to get sick or feel stress. If your "life force energy" is high, your experience is one of joy, happiness and health.

Rest days from exercise are a powerful *Winning Formula* in the recovery and rebuilding process. Rest days improve performance, protect a compromised immune system and prevent overtraining. Overtraining involves physical breakdown of muscles and joints, making it impossible to experience hypertrophy or strength gains, as well as hormonal disruption that creates imbalances in testosterone, cortisol and growth hormone.

Sound is vibration, an energy that moves within each of us long before we hear it. Each sound has its own unique frequency, vibration and wavelength. Sound therapy can help restore balance in areas where energy may be blocked.

In order to experience true healing on all levels, you must first be open to receive and desire the healing.

Aside from the various healing remedies, allowing and planning some sort of restoration and calmness into your lifestyle is incredibly healing. Discover people, things and places that nourish your soul and bring you back to center and help you heal.

Placing value and respect for rest and recovery comes with respecting the aging process and valuing yourself. This is especially true with exercise. Restoration is essential to hormonal balance and tissue regeneration. Relaxation and rest are desirable *Winning Formulas for Health, Vitality, Longevity and Fat Loss.*

Choose something that you genuinely enjoy doing and that you find mentally, spiritually and physically uplifting.

CHAPTER 4-6

WINNING FORMULAS FOR PHYSICAL EXERCISE

"We are made in the image of God and we need to put Spirit back into the equation when we want to improve our physical and our mental health."
~Bruce Lipton

Choose two *Winning Formulas* from the list below to implement this week. Write your two choices down on a piece of paper where they will be visible to you. Make copies. Keep them in several locations where you will see them.

- Be active with your children: Play outdoor games, family bike rides, hikes or walk to school.
- Bounce five to ten minutes daily on a mini-trampoline.
- Burn some essential oils in an aromatherapy diffuser.
- Choose a healing therapy that you're comfortable with.
- Do absolutely nothing for thirty minutes each day.
- Engage in exercise that's enjoyable – some form of movement you'll remain committed to.
- Exercise at a moderate pace four to five times a week for at least thirty minutes in duration.

- Exercise outside, especially away from the city, such as hiking, biking, etc.
- Find a workout partner.
- Learn one new exercise every week.
- Listen to relaxation tapes.
- Listen to your body.
- Maintain alignment of your spine, nerves and muscles with monthly chiropractic adjustments.
- Meditate and pray.
- Perform daily posture checks when you're driving, at your desk, standing in line at the store or anywhere.
- Practice stretching, yoga, Tai Chi or Qi Gong.
- Schedule a massage.
- Schedule an appointment with a qualified personal trainer.
- Schedule rest days from exercise.
- Spend time in nature.
- Take a road trip away from city life.
- Take a twenty to thirty minute walk every night after dinner.
- Understand limitations of your own body, despite what others may tell you.

- Use a stability ball for your desk chair instead of a regular chair. The stability ball activates the deep core musculature (your abs and back).

- When you awaken each morning, pay attention to your short, tight muscles. Take two to five minutes stretching those muscles.

CHAPTER 5

THE POWER OF SUPPLEMENTATION

"The purpose of life is joy."
~ The Dahli Lama

Supplementation is a topic of much confusion for many people. Supplements are integrated as a preventive ***Winning Formula*** to maintain or enhance ***Health, Vitality and Longevity and Fat Loss***. They are not a substitute for poor nutrition. On the contrary, nutritional supplementation is a powerful ***Winning Formula*** that offers various benefits to your health.

Few Americans get the minimum recommended amounts of vitamins and minerals from their diets. Even though each of us requires the same nutrients to be healthy, the amount of each nutrient can vary considerably due to individual factors such as: age, genetics, exposure to toxins, allergies and sensitivities, illness history, lifestyle, stress levels, symptom survey analysis, pregnancy, medications and personal health conditions.

People who smoke or consume alcohol, those with diabetes, women who take birth control pills along with pregnant women all have different nutritional requirements, as do those who suffer from allergies or who are ill.

Most individuals defer from incorporating nutritional supplements into their daily routine until they've been diagnosed with a serious illness.

According to the National Cancer Institute (NCI), "having a chronic medical condition such as cancer is the primary factor in a person's decision to use dietary supplements."

Poor quality of agriculture, environmental pollution, unhealthy diet habits, highly processed foods and extremely stressful lifestyles, as well as any person recovering from an illness, are just a few reasons people require additional support and protection. This is provided through nutritional supplementation.

Supplements act as catalysts for adequate nutrition. They are an important nutritional ally and a vital **Winning Formula** to any anti-aging program. Supplementation may improve quality of life in the elderly, acutely ill and patients who are hospitalized.

An article posted in the 2002 *Journal of the American Medical Association* states that "many of us require supplementation with vitamins; that suboptimal intake of certain nutrients is a risk factor for disease." Deficiencies of antioxidants, particularly vitamins A, C and E, are linked to an endless list of diseases. The article acknowledges that "the diets of the majority of Americans are not adequate in many of these nutrients and suggests supplementation."

Deficiencies of folic acid and vitamins B-6 and B-12 increase your risk for heart disease. Deficiencies in these vitamins increase your risk for colon and breast cancer, as well as neural tube defect in developing fetuses. Many elderly people have B-12 deficiencies. This affects the body's ability to deliver oxygen into each cell.

It can take weeks or months for a specific vitamin and/or mineral deficiency to eventually present itself. Individuals often notice a huge change in their health, or energy level, especially if they're supplementing with a particular nutrient they're deficient in. Vitamins rarely, if ever, make health issues worse.

According to a recent report from the *British Journal of Nutrition*, "men who use nutritional supplements demonstrated significantly reduced weight, lower body mass index and decreased fat mass than men who do not use nutritional supplements. These characteristics were also found among females, although they were less pronounced. Additionally, women who used supplements reported a reduction in appetite."

Choose to work with a health care practitioner who is trained in nutrition and natural therapies for guidance and recommendations for a supplement protocol specific to your individual requirements. Many individuals take herbs, vitamins and supplements without knowing or understanding what they're taking. Working with a qualified practitioner is not only safer, it is more effective.

Some herbs, for instance, taken on an empty stomach, work differently than when taken with food.

Dr. Harry Eidenier, Jr., Ph.D. quotes: *"Supplements should only be purchased from licensed/degreed and trained health care providers, professionals who have the education and clinical experience to provide you with practical information and reliable, non-toxic products."*

Quality control is relatively limited in the supplement and vitamin industry. Qualified and licensed practitioners are more likely to know which companies are high-quality and which formulas are superior. Biotics Research is a cutting-edge and innovative company. Biotics Research produces their supplements to pharmaceutical standards and has outstanding quality control. They specialize in the whole food approach to supplementation. Their supplements are food based. They use vegetable cultures which are rich in antioxidants. This ensures absorption of nutrients and proper tablet breakdown.

Winning Formula High-Quality Supplements:

- Biotics Research
- Designs for Health
- Pure Encapsulation
- Standard Process
- Thorne

CHAPTER 5-1

THE POWER OF SUPPLEMENTATION

DIGESTION AND HYDROCHLORIC ACID (HCl)

"The unhappiness in your life is not a result of the circumstances in your life, but a result from the conditioning of your mind."
~Eckhart Tolle

Digestion begins before you put food into your mouth, although this period is brief. Once you take a bite of food, your saliva starts to dissolve and soften the food. Chewing your food thoroughly is a *Winning Formula* that enhances digestion.

The best nutrition and supplement program won't do any good if your digestive system isn't working properly. You won't absorb, assimilate, metabolize and eliminate food molecules correctly. The worse your digestion, the more malnourished you become.

Hydrochloric acid (HCl) plays an important role in digestion and assimilation of nutrients. Your body's ability to absorb the nutrients you eat is an imperative *Winning Formula*. Difficulty with absorption can cause fatigue, skin rashes, migraine headaches and food intolerances.

Hydrochloric acid (HCl), which is produced by glands in your stomach, is necessary for the breakdown and digestion of many foods. Insufficient amounts of HCl make it more challenging for your body to digest protein. This can lead to indigestion.

HCl (hydrochloric acid) diminishes as you age. It is estimated that eighty percent of individuals over age sixty are deficient in hydrochloric acid, a condition known as hypochlorhydria.

Many people resort to antacids for indigestion and heartburn. Antacids contain aluminum which is toxic to your system. Heartburn is a signal that you're dehydrated.

You can determine if you require more hydrochloric acid with this simple test. Take a tablespoon of apple cider vinegar or lemon juice mixed in a small amount of water in the middle of your meal. If this resolves your indigestion, you require more stomach acid. If it makes your symptoms worse, you have too much acid. Although this is seldom the case, you would not take any supplements that contain HCl.

Many people with an insufficient amount of stomach acid have no obviously related symptoms. They're led to believe they are digesting properly when, in fact, they're not. HCl does not digest food on its own. It creates an environment in which digestion begins. Digestive enzymes help balance your body's pH. The food you eat and the supplements you take are absorbed at the cellular level when supplementing with digestive enzymes.

HCl is responsible for converting pepsinogen to pepsin, which begins breaking down proteins in your stomach. With limited HCl, pepsinogen isn't converted to pepsin and protein digestion fails. Consuming antacids inhibits optimal breakdown of proteins.

An additional action of HCl is to prevent infections. Most organisms that are ingested are completely destroyed by an acidic environment.

Without an adequate amount of HCl, your food and supplements are not broken down. Your body is less likely to assimilate and absorb these nutrients at the cellular level. A lack of HCl results in protein putrefication and carbohydrate fermentation in your body.

The *American Journal of Clinical Nutrition* reported that up to thirty percent of people over the age of sixty-five are unable to absorb vitamin B-12 and folic acid properly because they do not produce enough hydrochloric acid (HCl) and/or they suffer from an overgrowth of bacteria in the intestinal tract.

HCl requirements commonly exist with B-12 anemia. If you experience excessive stress, you end up creating a perfect environment for becoming hypo-hydrochloridic.

Proper digestion and absorption are fundamental *Winning Formulas* for optimal *Health, Vitality, Longevity and Fat Loss.*

Conditions of HCl deficiency or low stomach acid include:

- Acne, hives, eczema, psoriasis or other skin conditions
- Alcoholism
- Allergies
- Asthma
- Autoimmune diseases
- Bad breath and/or body odor
- Bloating and gas, especially after eating protein
- Candida, yeast infections or bacterial overgrowth of the stomach
- Drowsiness after meals
- Gallstones and gallbladder disorders
- H.pylori infection (caused by poor diet, nutrient deficiencies and toxin exposure)
- Heartburn
- Hypothyroidism
- Intestinal parasites
- Loss of taste for proteins
- Meal-related belching
- Migraines
- Mineral deficiencies
- Offensive smelling stools

- Osteoporosis
- Pancreatic dysfunction
- Rheumatoid arthritis
- Rosacea
- Sinus congestion
- Undigested food particles in stool
- Vertical lines in nails (white spots indicate ↓ zinc)
- Vitamin B-12 deficiency

Aside from supplementing with hydrochloric acid for digestive health, how you chew your food and the environment in which you eat are other factors that enhance or aggravate digestion. (See Chapter 2-5, Focus on Quality.)

The physical process of digestion starts in your mouth. Your saliva has enzymes that assist in digestion. Most people eat way too fast which stresses their digestive system. This creates problems of gas and bloating. Food is meant to be chewed and enjoyed, not inhaled. Improper chewing leads to poor absorption of nutrients, digestive complaints and promotes the growth of harmful bacteria in your digestive tract. Your body thinks you're dieting. It then proceeds to add body fat because it perceives famine at the cellular level imposed from inadequate nutrient absorption.

DO YOU HAVE A *WINNING* DIGESTIVE SYSTEM?

Do you experience one or more of the following?

Anal itching?

Belching or burping after meals?

Chronic yeast or fungal infections?

Constipation on a regular basis?

Excessive appetite or crave sweets?

Feel nauseated after taking supplements?

Frequent use of antibiotics (more than twice in three years)?

Gas after meals?

Greasy, poorly formed or foul smelling stools?

Headaches thirty to ninety minutes after eating?

Heartburn, indigestion, upset stomach, headache or acid reflux?

History of NSAIDs or other anti-inflammatories?

Less than one well-formed bowel movement daily?

Loose stools or diarrhea?

Lower abdominal bloating or distention after meals?

Poor appetite and/or feel worse after eating?

Regularly use antacids?

Sores on your tongue?

Undigested food particles in your stools?

Use of birth control pills or HRT (hormone replacement therapy)?

Use of prednisone or cortisone?

CHAPTER 5-2

THE POWER OF SUPPLEMENTATION

OMEGA-3 FISH OILS

"We are shaped by our thoughts; we become what we think. When the mind is pure, joy follows like a shadow that never leaves."
~Buddha

There is no disease known to man not remedied by fish oil. Fish oil is a ***Winning Formula*** supplement that can replace most expensive patented drugs and be just as effective without the negative side effects. It's not rocket science that long-term diet and nutrition habits have a direct affect on the way you look and feel. Recent studies show that proper supplementation, along with diet affects our thinking, moods and thought process.

Docosahexaenoic acid (DHA) is one of three omega-3 fatty acids crucial to human nutrition. The other two are alpha-linolenic acid (ALA) and eicosapentaenoic acid (EPA).

Your body converts ALA to EPA. EPA converts to DHA. Unfortunately, this conversion is not very efficient. Less than fifteen percent of ALA ends up as EPA. Research shows that less than five percent of EPA converts to DHA, under optimal conditions.

With the help of an enzyme, linoleic acid is converted to gamma-linoleic acid (GLA), an omega-6 fat. Very minimal amounts convert to GLA. Although some omega-6s are unhealthy when consumed in excess, primarily many vegetable oils and grains, GLA is a healthy omega-6. GLA is a powerful *Winning Formula* contributing to vibrant health and beautiful skin. (Refer to Chapter 2-3 for more on smart fats.)

GLA alters your body's production of hormone-like compounds called prostaglandins. Supplementing with GLA is beneficial for women who experience breast pain tenderness, although it may take three menstrual cycles before the effects are noticed. It can take up to eight months for the benefits of GLA supplemention to reach its full effect. GLA oil is especially useful for skin disorders. Dry skin may be an indication of GLA deficiency.

Your brain requires more omega-3 in the form of DHA as part of the natural anti-aging process for vitality and longevity.

Depression has been linked, in particular, to low levels of DHA. Low DHA results in a reduction of brain serotonin levels. The precise dose for treating depression can vary for each individual. Some experts recommend getting anywhere from five to fifteen grams of omega-3 fats three times daily. *(Fish oil supplements should never replace your medication. Always discuss any alternative treatment with your doctor first.)*

Aside from depression, low levels of DHA have been linked to bipolar disorder, schizophrenia, autism, memory loss, attention-deficit disorder, learning difficulties and bad moods. DHA protects your brain by feeding your brain cell membranes the appropriate type of fat.

Fish oil supplementation is a natural and safe *Winning Formula* alternative that may give support to bipolar disorder. The effects of fish oil for bipolar disorder have been tested in a recent study. The study revealed that "patients supplementing with fish oil experienced longer periods between symptoms versus those taking a placebo."

Dr. Eric Serrano, M.D. states, "Fish oil is the number one supplement guaranteed to lower elevated triglycerides."

NSAIDs are one of the principal pharmacological agents for treating arthritic pain and inflammation. However, concerns about the toxicity of NSAIDs have become increasingly well-known in recent years as gastrointestinal incidences of ulcers, perforation and bleeding are well documented.

Supplementation with cod liver oil, rich in omega-3 fatty acids, was found to alleviate pain and inflammation far superior to NSAIDs. Thus, individuals suffering with rheumatoid arthritis reduced or completely eliminated their dosages of non-steroidal anti-inflammatory drugs (NSAIDs) when supplementing with cod liver oil.

It is imperative to include "essential" fatty acids in your diet. These fats cannot be manufactured by your body.

As stated in Chapter 2-3, aside from supplements, oily fish such as wild salmon is a nourishing source of DHA. Vegetarians must ensure they supplement daily with high-grade fish oil. Vegans can obtain DHA from chia, micro-algae, seaweed, ground flax seed and various nuts and seeds. Flaxseed may contain many health-promoting benefits, although flaxseed does not provide you with adequate amounts of EPA and DHA.

DHA, the most dominant essential fatty acid in the brain, is crucial to fetal and infant brain, eyes and nervous system development. After birth, omega-3 levels depend on the infant's innate lipid metabolism and dietary intake from breast milk. Although EPA and DHA are prominent ingredients in breast milk, many formulas do not contain these nutrients. In recent years, manufactured DHA has been added to infant formulas. Infants experience side effects when fed formula with these manufactured oils. Breast feeding is the healthiest way to feed a human infant.

The need for DHA increases dramatically in the third trimester of fetal life and the first two years of childhood. This is a critical period of rapid brain growth and central nervous system development.

In a randomized study involving pregnant women, "daily supplementation with DHA (docosahexaenoic acid, 400 mg/d) from sixteen weeks of gestation until delivery was found to be associated with superior visual acuity in infants at sixty days of age as compared to infants born to women who received a placebo."

Fish oil may be equally important to the elderly as it is to infants. The American Heart Association has endorsed omega-3 fatty acids as a preventative measure against heart disease. Fish oil has long been advocated as an affordable supplement to prevent or at least delay Alzheimer's disease. Low omega-3 fatty acid levels were found to be associated with dementia.

Realistically, suggesting dietary recommendations to eat fish as your primary source of fish oil, EPA/DHA, is threatened by the fact that quality fish have become rather expensive. Quality fish is difficult to come across. Wild salmon and other species that are not contaminated with mercury or other pollutants are increasingly restricted and shrinking in supply.

Researchers with the Southern California Coastal Water Research Project discovered that two-thirds of some species of fish examined from coastal waters off Los Angeles and Orange Counties possess both male and female reproductive organs. The seafloor sediment in these areas is contaminated with estrogenic chemicals from wastewater sewage generated by nine million inhabitants of coastal cities.

High-grade fish oil supplements contain fewer toxins and pollutants than fish. Various laboratory examinations found pharmaceutical fish oil supplements to be free of mercury and other contaminants. This is related to the fact that mercury accumulates in the muscle tissue versus the fat tissue. When the fish oils are processed, toxins are removed.

Some individuals complain of "fish burps" or "belching" when they supplement with fish oils. If this occurs, it indicates your body is not emulsifying the oils, indicating gallbladder and liver support is required. Additionally, you may be supplementing with a low-grade brand of fish oil. If, upon switching to a higher-quality, pharmaceutical-grade fish oil the belching continues, this implies a malfunctioning digestive system. Consider supplementing with HCl in the middle of your meal. Doing so often alleviates the belching. (See Chapter 5-1.) Other factors to consider are your gallbladder. Your gallbladder may require supplemental support, a cleanse or flush. Your gallbladder releases a substance called bile, which assists in the digestion of fats.

Most Americans consume an extraordinary amount of omega-6 foods in their diets. This causes an imbalanced ratio of omega-6 to omega-3 (See Chapter 2-3.) Excess intake of omega-6 foods lead to increased inflammation, elevated blood pressure, an irritated digestive tract, decreased immunity, sterility, cancer and extra body weight.

Indications of essential fatty acid insufficiency include:

- Allergies (i.e.: eczema/asthma/hay fever/hives)
- Cotton mouth/throat
- Cracks on heels and/or peeling fingertips
- Crave fats/fatty foods
- Dandruff or cradle cap
- Depression
- Dry eyes, hair and/or skin
- Dull nails - lack of surface shine
- Elevated triglycerides
- Excessive ear wax build-up
- Extreme thirst
- Hair loss
- Inadequate vaginal lubrication
- Learning disabilities
- Menstrual cramps
- Patchy dullness and/or color variation of skin
- Premenstrual breast pain/tenderness
- Quilted appearance of skin (i.e.: legs)
- Slow-growing fingernails

- Small bumps on back of upper arms
- Soft, fraying, splitting or brittle fingernails
- Stiff, achy or painful joints
- Thick or cracked calluses
- Weight gain (increased body fat)

In a placebo-controlled, double-blind, parallel design study, exercisers were given either 8 one gram capsules per day of olive oil (placebo) or fish oil for a period of eight weeks. Fish oil was found to reduce heart rate and oxygen consumption during exercise without a decrement in performance. Omega-3 fatty acids also have beneficial effects on thermogenesis (fat burning).

Fish oil is one of the most effective supplements for reducing inflammation and insulin resistance.

Individuals that have elevated plasma levels of high-sensitivity C-reactive protein (hs-CRP, a marker of low-grade sustained inflammation) benefit from omega-3 supplementation. Elevated CRP was found to be inversely associated with total omega-3 fatty acids, EPA, and DPA levels.

Other nutrients that have demonstrated effects in suppressing chronic inflammation and insulin resistance include: chromium, vitamin D, curcumin, tumeric, boswelia, magnesium, Gymnema Sylvestre, cinnamon, resveratrol and polyphenols found in cocoa, green tea and apples.

Fish oils are inexpensive and devoid of the dangerous side effects of prescription drugs. Fish oil is best taken with extra vitamin E (as mixed tocopherols).

Vitamin E prevents the oils from oxidizing too quickly in your body. Always take your fish oil with food, preferably at the end of your meal.

High-grade *Winning Formula* brands of fish oil include:

- Biotics Research
- Designs for Health
- Nordic Naturals
- Pure Encapsulation
- Thorne

Benefits of Omega-3 Fish Oils Include:

- # 1 supplement for depression, bi-polar, diabetes and ADHD
- ↓ inflammation and symptoms of inflammatory diseases such as arthritis
- Cardiovascular disease prevention (50% reduction)
- Clearer skin, stronger nails, shinier hair
- Corrects gut dysfunction
- Decreased LDL cholesterol and lowers triglycerides

- Healthy development for infants, boosting brain power
- Helps balance hormones and ↓ PMS symptoms
- Improved brain function
- Improved Lupus symptoms
- Increased emotional well-being
- Lower risk of breast and prostate cancer
- Mood stabilization in manic-depressive and bi-polar

- Natural anti-inflammatory
- Promotes fat loss
- Protect us from viruses and yeasts
- Protects liver from alcohol and other toxins such as Tylenol
- Reduced growth and size of tumors
- Regulates insulin levels; improves insulin sensitivity and helps insulin resistant and diabetic individuals

CHAPTER 5-3

THE POWER OF SUPPLEMENTATION

MULTIPLE VITAMIN AND VITAMIN D

"Give no deadly medicine to anyone."
~Hippocrates

The best health insurance you can buy is supplementing with a high-quality, *Winning Formula,* multi vitamin. Just a century ago, our food contained all the nutrients our bodies required to function optimally. Nowadays, it's impossible to find adequate levels of nutrients in our foods alone.

Do you need supplements? If you eat wild, fresh, organic, local, non-genetically modified food grown in nutrient-rich soils, breathe only fresh unpolluted air, drink only pure, clean water, sleep eight hours a night, move your body every day, and are free from chronic stress and exposure to environmental toxins, you may not need supplements. For the rest of us, supplements are a necessity.

Insufficient vitamin and mineral levels predispose you to degenerative diseases. In addition, vitamin and mineral deficiencies may lead to symptoms of ADD and ADHD. Taking a good quality multivitamin-mineral supplement every day is a basic *Winning Formula* to build a foundation of good health and is invaluable in warding off life-threatening diseases.

In 2002 the *Journal of the American Medical Association* reported a relationship between chronic disease and vitamin intake, recommending that all adults take a multi-vitamin daily because the absence of these vitamins in their foods places them at risk for cancer, cardiovascular disease and osteoporosis. It's evident that vitamins and minerals are essential for brain function and health.

Not all multivitamins are equal or designed to improve overall health. The majority of the better quality supplement companies sell directly to licensed practitioners only. If you have a doctor who is familiar with natural health and nutrition, he or she is your ultimate source from which to purchase your supplements.

Only high-quality supplements provide your cells with the best nutrition for function and performance. Commercially available vitamins are made with synthetic, inactive ingredients that interfere with absorption. Poor quality, synthetic supplements hinder health due to the added dyes, coloring, binders and fillers. Quality supplements are easier for your body to absorb than most vitamins found in health food or discount stores.

A key *Winning Formula* regarding your multivitamin – take it with food, preferably at the end of your meal.

The "sunshine vitamin," also known as vitamin D has been associated with endless health benefits so that it may become the "nutrient of the decade." Vitamin D deficiency is now recognized as a pandemic. Extensive research over the past twenty years documents a remarkable "paradigm shift" in understanding vitamin D. Unlike other vitamins, vitamin D is a hormone precursor.

While federal officials have resisted increasing the daily recommended level of vitamin D out of fears of overdose toxicity, mounting evidence suggests that the currently recommended intake levels are not adequate to prevent the serious diseases linked to low vitamin D levels.

One study on people living beyond age ninety revealed that these people had two things in their favor: "a functional thyroid and adequate levels of vitamin D."

In 2003 Mayo Clinic acknowledged vitamin D deficiency as a "cause of fatigue, feelings of heaviness in the legs and chronic and vague musculoskeletal pain." Lower concentrations of 25(OH)D, also called 25-hydroxyvitamin D, are associated with significant back pain in older women. A study from the University of Minnesota revealed that "ninety-three percent of their 150 study subjects were deficient in vitamin D. The worst vitamin D deficiencies were found in women of child-bearing age. Vitamin D deficiency is an epidemic in pregnant women. Deficiencies cause permanent injury to fetal brains."

Another study involving 291 elderly men revealed that "only two of the subjects had normal vitamin D levels."

A lack of vitamin D can initiate, precipitate and exacerbate a host of health disorders. Symptoms may manifest as inflammatory diseases, bone metabolism disorders, infectious diseases and immunological imbalances. One of the major signs of vitamin D deficiency is bone pain, technically referred to as osteomalacia.

Vitamin D insufficiency, which is quite prevalent among obese adolescents, is more common among older adolescents and those with higher systolic blood pressure and lower HDL cholesterol levels. Because of the many vitamin D receptors in the brain, it has been discovered that vitamin D plays a very important role in maintaining and achieving a healthy mind.

Common reasons for reduced vitamin D levels include: aging, cancer (breast, bowel, prostate), dark skin, fat malabsorption, fractures, free radical disease, limited sun exposure and use of sunscreen, obesity, parathyroid dysfunction, use of anticonvulsant medications and kidney, liver and other organ dysfunction.

Very few foods naturally contain vitamin D. Foods that are fortified with vitamin D are often inadequate to satisfy either a child's or an adult's vitamin D requirement. Vitamin D is found in wild-caught oily fish such as salmon, mackerel, bluefish, catfish, sardines and tuna or cod liver oil, sun-dried Shitake mushrooms, raw milk and eggs.

Very small amounts of vitamin D are found in fortified foods, such as some orange juices, milk and some cereals. Utilization of vitamin D by your body can be inhibited by an excessive consumption of cereal grains.

Three options exist for treatment of vitamin D deficiency – sunlight, artificial UVB light and vitamin D3 supplementation.

The lab test for vitamin D status is 25(OH)D, also called 25-hydroxyvitamin D. It is an inexpensive test worth checking.

Pregnant women or women considering pregnancy should have their vitamin D levels checked every three months. Professor Neil Binkley, a Vitamin D researcher at the University of Wisconsin states, "The body doesn't start storing cholecalciferol (D3) until levels reach 50 ng/mL." This means that current "normal" lab values showing serum concentration at 20-56 ng/mL are inappropriately low to optimize health. Dr. Harry Eidenier, Jr., Ph.D. affirms, "The optimal 25(OH)D value is 60-100 ng/mL."

Researchers from Finland found that people who had the highest blood levels of vitamin D were seventy-two percent less likely to develop diabetes than those with the lowest levels.

Current data suggests vitamin D is more important than calcium for prevention of factures. Vitamin D helps normalize calcium metabolism which has a very positive effect on your bones and teeth.

Another study revealed that "fifty percent of colon cancer incidence in North America could be prevented by maintaining adequate levels of vitamin D." Fr̶ ̶t̶h̶e̶r̶m̶o̶r̶e̶ ̶t̶h̶e̶ ̶s̶t̶u̶d̶y̶ projects a "thirty percent reduction in bre̶ in North America with lifelong maintenanc̶ ̶ ̶levels equal to, or above 42 ng/mL."

Vitamin D can also be synthe̶ body upon exposure to sunlight.

Vitamin D is a *Winning Formula* found to:
• Be a natural solution for high blood pressure
• Be beneficial for age related diseases
• Enhance immunity
• Increase cognitive performance
• Lower your risk of cancer
• Lower your risk of diabetes
• Prevent autoimmune conditions
• Protect against inflammation and chronic back pain
• Provide cardiovascular protection
• Reduce tumor growth
• Reduce your risk of multiple sclerosis
• Strengthen bones

Stress of any sort causes your body to use up available nutrients at a faster than normal pace. Select a multi-vitamin specific to your personal circumstances and lifestyle as a *Winning Formula*.

The result of a placebo controlled study suggests that "a single 1000 milligram dose of vitamin C prior to exercise may prevent exercise-induced lipid peroxidation and muscle damage."

Alcohol and drugs, such as aspirin and birth control pills may reduce vitamin C levels in your body. An alarming fifteen tons of aspirin are consumed daily by Americans. Intake of aspirin, Tylenol or other NSAID (non-steroidal anti-inflammatory drug) drugs will reduce pain, HOWEVER, at the risk of increasing oxidative stress and organ damage. Instead of speeding recovery from muscular injury, ingestion of NSAIDs may actually slow the process for several days as protein synthesis (tissue healing) is delayed. Approximately 16,500 ulcer-related complicated deaths occur in the United States alone from the use of NSAIDs. In fact, use of NSAIDs, steroids, antacids and antibiotics are some of the greatest contributors to digestive distress and leaky gut syndrome.

Inflammation can be prevented or reduced by adding more fruits and vegetables to your diet, increasing intake of omega-3 fats and reducing intake of trans fats and simple carbohydrates. Some herbs and phytochemicals shown to reduce inflammation include curcumin, ginger, rosemary and basil.

Be informed! Be empowered! Take control and responsibility.

Adverse side effects from OTC aspirin and NSAIDs include:

- Bleeding
- Death
- Depression
- Edema
- Headaches

- Increased risk for ulcers
- Increased intestinal permeability and gastric distress
- Irritation to the bowel lining
- Kidney failure
- Liver stress

- Nausea
- Reye's syndrome
- Shortness of breath
- Sleep disturbances

In addition, NSAIDs will actually encourage pain, arthritis and inflammation – the very reason one takes NSAID to begin with.

Remember, all drugs have side effects, are toxic to your body and cause stress to your organs.

238

CHAPTER 5-4

THE POWER OF SUPPLEMENTATION

INTESTINAL HEALTH AND PROBIOTICS

"Raise yourself to the level of energy where you are the light you seek, where you are the happiness you desire, where you are the love you feel is missing, where you are the unlimited abundance you crave."
~Dr. Wayne Dyer

Did you know that your gut and digestive system influence the health of your body? Your natural defense system – your immune system – is affected by the bacteria in your gut.

When you hear the word "bacteria" you may imagine something unpleasant. Not all bacteria are considered to be harmful. Good bacteria live and thrive in your intestines and the vagina. They protect you against the invasion and growth of harmful bacteria. There are up to four pounds of bacteria in the human intestinal tract consisting of both healthy and unhealthy bacteria. Bacteria (flora) in your bowels outnumber the cells in your body by 10:1.

An overload of unhealthy bacteria can cause infections, chronic health problems and a wide range of disease.

A beneficial bacterium in your body creates lactase which is an enzyme that works to break down lactose (milk sugar) into simple sugars that your body can digest. You may have heard of the term "lactose-intolerant." This individual does not produce the lactase enzyme. Probiotics would be highly beneficial for these individuals.

The term probiotic literally means "to promote life." Probiotics are active-living, beneficial micro-organisms such as lactobacillus, streptococcus, acidophilus, bulgaricus, casei, thermophilus and bifidobacteria. They are located in your intestinal tract. Probiotics are supplements that balance and re-establish healthy flora in your body.

According to research in the *Proceedings of the Nutrition Society* (2007, Volume 66) "supplementing with probiotics can improve antioxidant status. Thereby, probiotics protect your body against oxidative stress." Oxidative stress is a threat to your health and promotes aging. It can trigger feelings of fatigue. Oxidative stress can be the root cause of serious health conditions such as heart disease and cancer.

Factors that cause imbalances of bacteria in your body:

- Alcohol consumption
- Antibiotic use
- Birth control pills
- Chemically-altered foods
- Diabetes

- Environmental pollution
- Estrogen replacement therapy
- Inadequate fiber intake
- Poor immune function

- Reduced HCl (See Chapter 5-1.)
- Rheumatoid arthritis
- Slow bowel transit time
- Steroid drugs
- Stress

The flora in your digestive system contributes to weight management. Seventy percent of your immune system is located in your digestive system. When you consume sugar, your immune system is suppressed for up to eight hours afterwards.

One of the most crucial *Winning Formula* actions you can implement to influence healthy flora in your digestive system is to eliminate all sugars and refined grains. These foods are the perfect food source for yeast and parasites. Sugar and refined carbohydrates feed the harmful bacteria in your gut and colon, which promote disease. When the unhealthy bacteria initiate growth, it doubles approximately every twenty minutes.

Research suggests that women with endometriosis may have bacterial or yeast over-growth in their gastrointestinal tract which will aggravate bloating, stomach pain, diarrhea and/or constipation. In one study conducted at the Women's Hospital of Texas in Houston, "forty out of fifty women studied had excessive levels of bacteria in their gastrointestinal tract."

Alcoholic livers may benefit from probiotic supplementation. A study published in *The Journal of Hepatology* found that "patients who supplemented with probiotics noted improvements in the immune function of their white blood cells."

Probiotics encourage *Winning Formula* health benefits such as:

- A powerful boost to your immune system
- Avoidance of yeast and urinary infections
- Breakdown of xenoestrogens and toxins
- Decreased risk of diverticulitis, inflammatory bowel disease and irritable bowel syndrome
- Eliminates diarrhea by enhancing digestion of fats and proteins
- Encourages a healthy functioning digestive system by maximizing food assimilation.
- Excellent to supplement with throughout pregnancy and breastfeeding for development of infants' immune system
- Helps to produce vitamin K in the body
- Improved neurocognitive function for chronic fatigue
- Inhibits harmful bacteria
- Nourishes the lining of your colon
- Plays a key role in preventing osteoporosis
- Prevents side effects from antibiotics restoring healthy flora
- Produces vitamins, such as folic acid and B-12
- Reduces blood fats/cholesterol

Probiotics are available as capsules, tablets or powder. Foods that contain probiotics include cultured, fermented yogurt, kefir and raw sauerkraut. Chicory root is a natural source of prebiotics known as FOS.

Probiotics are healing for your gut. They're effective for treating yeast infections. Inflammation of the stomach can feel like chest or neck pain. Intestinal inflammation can appear as low back pain.

In addition to probiotics, the following are also healing *Winning Formulas* for your gut and intestinal tract:

- Fresh cabbage juice
- Gamma oryzanol
- Ginger tea
- High-dose fish oil
- L-glutamine (heals the gut and regulates insulin resistance)
- Liquid aloe Vera juice
- Slippery elm tea

A healthy gut equals a healthy person!

CHAPTER 5-5

THE POWER OF SUPPLEMENTATION

MAGNESIUM

"If we could give every individual the right amount of nourishment and exercise, not too little and not too much, we would have found the safest way to health."

~Hippocrates

Magnesium is the fourth most abundant mineral in your body. It's a building block for cellular physiology. Magnesium is considered the "anti-stress" mineral and is known as nature's muscle relaxer. It is an essential **Winning Formula** mineral for quality health.

Magnesium is a vital cofactor in over 300 chemical reactions in your body. It's found in tissues with high metabolic activity. Magnesium is important for ATP synthesis (cellular energy). Your heart, liver, brain and kidney contain the highest intracellular concentrations of magnesium. Without adequate magnesium, your body accumulates toxins and acid residues. This causes your body to degenerate and prematurely age.

Magnesium is a *Winning Formula* for:

- Alcoholics
- Allergies
- Asthma
- Atherosclerosis
- Caffeine withdraw
- Cardiac stress

- Chronic Fatigue Syndrome
- Constipation
- Diabetes
- Fibromyalgia
- Gluten-sensitivity
- Hypertension

- Hypoglycemia
- Kidney and gallstones
- Osteoporosis (synergist to calcium)
- Muscle cramps (Charley horses)
- PMS – mood swings and breast tenderness
- Promotes estrogen detoxification
- Psychological stress

Magnesium deficiency is very common, especially in the elderly. In addition, deficiency is likely in people who use alcohol, caffeine, excessive sugar, hypertension medication, birth control pills and those addicted to sleep aids. Individuals who experience a high-stress lifestyle tend to have insufficient levels of magnesium.

Deficiency in magnesium may present as chocolate cravings, difficulty relaxing, problems falling asleep, constipation and an inability to metabolize estrogen in the liver.

According to a research review from Northwestern University, "magnesium was found to increase HDL cholesterol and decrease triglycerides."

Magnesium inhibits the absorption of aluminum to assist in the prevention of Alzheimer's disease. Magnesium also protects your cells from absorbing other toxic heavy metals such as mercury, lead, cadmium, beryllium and nickel.

Magnesium is essential for strong, healthy bones at all stages of life. Approximately fifty percent of total body magnesium is found in bone. Magnesium is a vital *Winning Formula* to guard against osteoporosis. In two separate studies published in the *American Journal of Clinical Nutrition,* magnesium deficiency was found to be associated with abnormal bone calcification. Both studies revealed that "the higher the intake of magnesium, the higher the level of bone mineral density." Magnesium is a synergist for calcium and vitamin D absorption.

Calcium and magnesium are opposites in their effects on your body. Calcium causes muscles to contract, while magnesium helps them relax. Usually the more inflexible and rigid your body is the less calcium but more magnesium you need. Leg cramping (Charley horses) and your toes turning up are indicators of magnesium deficiency.

Migraine headaches are one of the most painful and debilitating conditions you may experience. Magnesium has been found to reduce the frequency and severity of migraine headaches. Fifty percent of individuals who suffer with migraines are magnesium-deficient. Magnesium works by relaxing blood vessels in the brain and inhibiting the ability of calcium to constrict blood vessels. People with a low intake of magnesium in their diet may be at greater risk for stroke.

Alcohol consumption has always been known to deplete magnesium from your body. The more alcohol one consumes the lower their magnesium levels. Magnesium is one of the first supplements given to alcoholics when they eliminate alcohol and detoxify their systems.

Food sources of magnesium include: cocoa powder, dark chocolate (high in flavonoids), legumes, nuts and seeds, meat and seafood, spinach and unprocessed, whole grains such as millet, buckwheat and quinoa.

Magnesium supplementation is inexpensive and convenient. For optimal absorption, magnesium is best taken before bedtime, away from food, when little or no fat is present in the gastrointestinal tract. Magnesium will bind with available fat which prevents absorption of both, the fat and the magnesium.

While the recommended daily allowance of magnesium is 420 mg/day for men and 320 mg/day for women, many experts recommend adults consume at least 600 to 1000 mg/day because the absorption rate for magnesium is so low. Extra-large doses of magnesium may cause loose stools.

The amount of magnesium intake must factor your calcium intake. The ratio of calcium to magnesium should be 1:1. Many individuals supplement excessively with calcium overlooking magnesium and vitamin D. Magnesium is crucial in your body's ability to absorb calcium.

Dr. Mark Sircus, author of *Winning the War on Cancer,* states that "calcium requirements for men and women are lower than previously estimated."

Excessive levels of calcium cause adverse side effects which include: hypertension and stroke, arthritic joint degeneration, kidney stones, mood and depressive disorders as well as mineral deficiencies.

According to Dr. Jerry Aikawa, "magnesium is the most important mineral to man and all living organisms."

Constipation

Constipation is a serious, unspoken problem rampant in the United States. Laxatives are the third best selling item at drug stores.

Normal bowel transit time is twenty-four to forty-eight hours. From a functional perspective, an individual is considered constipated if a day passes without a bowel movement. Constipation leads to an accumulation of toxins in your body. Many experts agree that ninety percent of all disease starts in the bowel. If you experience constipation, first consider changing your diet and drinking an adequate amount of water.

Fried and processed foods, sugar, peanut butter and dairy products cause constipation. Other common causes for constipation include: dehydration, lack of dietary fiber, magnesium deficiency, HCl deficiency, lack of exercise, antidepressants, bile congestion with a need for bile salts, gut dysbiosis, low thyroid function, stress and unresolved emotional issues.

Winning Formulas to reduce or alleviate constipation:

- Aloe Vera juice in the morning
- Before bedtime, eat half of a raw potato with Celtic sea salt
- Eat organic, cooked rhubarb
- Deep, full breathing
- Drinking an adequate amount of water
- Eliminating dairy products
- High fiber diet
- Magnesium up to bowel tolerance
- One tablespoon of sesame oil before bedtime
- Yoga, Qi Gong and Tai Chi

CHAPTER 5-6

WINNING FORMULAS FOR SUPPLEMENTATION

"Healing requires taking action. It is not a passive event. When a person seeks to see more, healing is inevitable."
~Caroline Myss

- Always take your multi-vitamin and fish oil with food – immediately after your meal.
- Avoid iron-deficiency anemia – include iron-rich foods and consider a high-quality fish oil and multi-vitamin.
- Be consistent taking supplements.
- Consider HCl in the middle of your meal.
- Consider quality, pharmaceutical supplements that contain no dyes, colors and/or binding ingredients.
- Consider supplementing with GLA in the form of borage oil or evening primrose oil if you experience breast tenderness or suffer from dry skin.
- Consider supplementing with magnesium at bedtime – away from food.
- Discuss all supplements you take with your health practitioner.

- Eliminate foods that cause constipation.

- For insulin resistance or type II diabetes, consider cod liver oil, lipoic acid and various botanicals such as fenugreek, Gymnema sylvestre, bitter gourd, banaba and cinnamon

- Get twenty minutes of sunlight daily for natural vitamin D.

- If on blood pressure or cholesterol medication, seek the advice of a naturopathic medical doctor for healthier alternatives.

- If on thyroid medication, take thyroid medication one to two hours away from iron or vitamin C.

- If you supplement with calcium, make sure you include magnesium supplementation – ideal ratio is 1:1.

- If you're a vegetarian, consider high-grade fish oil, a multi-vitamin with iron and sublingual B-12.

- Obtain current lab testing. (See pages 149-150 for a complete list of suggested tests.)

- Organize your supplements for the day. Get a pill box to keep in your purse or briefcase.

- Seek the assistance from a health practitioner for a supplement protocol specific to you, amounts to be taken and the ideal time to take your particular supplements.

- Test for optimal vitamin D values. Consider vitamin D supplementation.

See page 251 for *Winning Formulas* to alleviate constipation.

CHAPTER 6

IMPLEMENTING *THE POWER OF 4*
Your *Winning Formulas for Health, Vitality, Longevity and Fat Loss*

"Change your thoughts – change your life."
~Wayne Dyer

You've been enlightened with a vast amount of information after reading **THE POWER OF 4.** Now it's time to implement what you've learned. You have the power and potential to put your knowledge into action. Go back and re-read Chapter 1-2, "Goal Setting: Be the Change." Start simple. As stated, each week you will select two *Winning Formulas* for your intended action.

Pay attention to how you feel every week, physically and emotionally. As you eliminate toxic foods, products and people, you may experience what is called the "healing crisis." A healing crisis is any wide range of symptoms that may occur during the course of healing. The onset of these symptoms is very rapid. The worst of the symptoms may last as little as a few hours or as long as several days. The longer the symptoms last, the stronger your personal healing crisis. These symptoms are the effects of detoxification. This is a positive sign that healing is taking place.

Your body is working to eliminate its storage of toxins – materials that have been collected in your colon, tissues and individual cells. When the symptoms disappear, you will feel amazing!

Physical symptoms may present as irritability, fatigue, headaches, skin rashes, cravings and/or nausea. Possible emotional reactions may include feelings of deprivation, distress and fear.

Focus on becoming as healthy as possible. Make choices based on what will make you healthier today, tomorrow and for the rest of your life. Change does not happen overnight. Practice patience. Keep the faith. Empower and inspire others by sharing *THE POWER OF 4* with your friends, family and co-workers. Form a *POWER OF 4* support group. Be an active participant in your life. You now have the knowledge to change your body and transform your life!

THE POWER OF 4 is your opportunity to experience *Health, Vitality, Longevity and Fat Loss!*

Thank you for reading *THE POWER OF 4.*
I personally wish you abundance and success.
Health, Vitality, Longevity and Fat Loss are yours!
With love and gratitude,

Paula Owens

RESOURCES

Audio version of *THE POWER OF 4*
www.PaulaOwens.com

Supplements
To purchase any of the supplements covered in this book, please contact Paula Owens.
Email: Paula@PaulaOwens.com
Website: www.PaulaOwens.com

Labs:
- Genova Labs
- Doctor's Data

Grass-Fed Beef
- Pacific Village – Entirely grass-fed cattle since 2002
  www.newseasonsmarket.com

- Diamond Organics
  www.diamondorganics.com

- Grassland Beef
  www.grasslandbeef.com

Informative Websites

www.bioticsresearch.com

www.ccnh.edu

www.charlespoliquin.com

www.ewg.org

www.gotmercury.org

www.notmilk.com

www.organic-center.org

www.ppnf.org

www.realmilk.com

www.safecosmetics.org

www.soyonlineservice.co.nz

www.totalfitness.net

www.westonaprice.org

REFERENCES

CHAPTER ONE REFERENCES

Wijndaele K, Duvigneaud N, et al. (2007). Sedentary behavior, physical activity and a continuous metabolic syndrome risk score in adults, *European Journal of Clinical Nutrition.*

Lutsey PL, Steffen LM, Stevens J. (2008).Dietary intake and the development of the metabolic syndrome. *Circulation.* 117(6): 754-61.

Wang Y, Beydoun MA. The obesity epidemic in the United States; gender, age, socioeconomic, racial/ethnic and geographic characteristics. (2007). *Epidemiologic Reviews.* 29: 6-28.

Physicians and the Pharmaceutical Industry, *JAMA.* January 19, 2000.

Conscientiousness and the incidence of Alzheimer disease and mild cognitive impairment. Wilson RS, Schneider JA, et al, *Arch Gen Psychiatry,* 2007; 64(10): 1204-12.

The Ecologist, October, 2000.

Oorganic-center.org

Health Letter, 1989:5(7):1-5.

2000. Brostoff, J and Gamlin, L. Food Allergies and Food Intolerance. Inner Traditions   Intl Ltd.

Cerami, A., Vlassara, H., and Brownlee, M. Glucose and aging. *Scientific American.* May 1987:90.

Lee, A. T. and Cerami, A. The role of glycation in aging. *Annals of the New York Academy of Science;* 663:63-67.

Abrahamson, E. and Peget, *A. Body, mind and sugar.* New York: Avon, 1977.

Keen, H., et al. Nutrient Intake, Adiposity and diabetes. *British Medical Journal.* 1989; 655-658.

Environmental Health Perspectives. 111(7). June 2003. http://www.pubmedcentral.nih.gov.

Association between obesity and cancer incidence. Kjaer D, Horvath-Puho E, et al, BJOG, 2007 Nov 12. http://www.jrussellshealth.org/pestsfacts.html

*Science Direct:*10.1016/j.physletb.2003.10.071.

Shim, Y.K. et al., "Parental Exposure to Pesticides and Childhood Brian Cancer: United States Atlantic Coast Childhood Brian Cancer Study," *Environmental Health Perspectives,*

Geiser, M. (2003) The wonders of whey protein. *NSCA Performance Training Journal* 2, 13-15.

CHAPTER TWO REFERENCES

Lancet. (2007). Food additives and hyperactive behavior in 3-year-old and 8/9-year-old children in the community.

Launer JL, Ross GW, Petrovich H,et al Midlife blood pressure ad dementia: the Honolulu-Asia aging study. Neurobiol Aging 2000;21:49-55

American Chemical Society (2007, August 23). Soda Warning? High-fructose corn syrup linked to diabetes.

Blaylock, Russell L. (1997). *Excitotoxins.*

University of Barcelona (2007, March 16). Fructose-sweetened beverages increases risk of obesity in rats.

American Psychological Association (2008, February 11). Artificial sweeteners linked to weight gain.

Haas, Elson (1992). *Staying Healthy with Nutrition.*

Meyerowitz, Steve. (2001). *Water, the Ultimate Cure.*

Batmanghelidj, F. (1997). *Your Body's Many Cries for Water.*

Haas, Elson (1992). *Staying Healthy with Nutrition.*

University of Cincinnati (2008, February 4). Plastic bottles release potentially harmful chemicals (Bisphenol A) after contact with hot liquids. *Science Daily.* Retrieved March 21, 2008. http://www.sciencedaily.com releases/2008/01/080130092108.htm.

Bailey A.B., Ph. D., Chemistry Review, Food and Drug Administration. 1996. Cumulative exposure estimated for bisphenol A (BPA), individually for adults and infants from its use in epoxy-based can coatings and polycarbonate (PC) Articles Branch, HFS-245. P. D. G. Diachenki, Division of Product Manufacture and Use, HGS-245.

Brotons JA, Olea-Serrano MF, Villalobos M, Pedraza V, Olea N. 1995. Xenoestrogens released from lacquer coatings in food cans. *Environ Health Perspect* 103: 608-12.

Howdeshell, K, AK Hotchkiss, KA Thayer, JG Vandenbergh and FS vom Saal. 1999. Plastic bisphenol A speeds growth and puberty. *Nature* 401: 762-764.

Takeuchi T, Tsutsumi O, Ikezuki Y, Takai Y, Taketani Y. 2004. Positive relationship between androgen and the endocrine disruptor, bisphenol A, in normal women and women with ovarian dysfunction. *Endocr J* 51(2): 165-9.

Timms BG, Howdeshell KL, Barton L, Bradley S, Richter CA, vom Saal FS. 2005. Estrogenic chemicals in plastic and oral contraceptives disrupt development of the fetal mouse prostate and urethra. *Proceedings of the National Academy of Sciences of the United States of America* 102(19): 7014-9.

Thomson, B. M. and P. R. Grounds (2005). Bisphenol A in canned foods in New Zealand: an exposure assessment. *Food Addit Contam* 22(1): 65-72.

www.westonaprice.org/women/natural_protection.html

FoodNavigator.com Oct, 2007.

http://www.jrussellshealth.org/microwaves.html#plastic

Our oceans are turning into plastics...are we? 2007. www.bestlifeonline.com/cms/publish/health.

Fructose consumption and the risk of kidney stones. (2007). *Kidney Int.*

C. Van Loveren, *European Journal of Pediatric Dentistry*, Feb, 2000.

Association of urinary bisphenol A concentration with medical disorders and laboratory abnormalities in adults," Lang IA, Galloway TS, et al, JAMA, 2008; 300(11): 1303-10.

Weight-loss diet that includes consumption of medium-chain triacylglycerol oil leads to a greater rate of weight and fat mass loss than does olive oil. *Am J Clin Nutr* (2008). 87 621-626. http://www.ajcn.org/cgi/content/abstract/87/3/621.

Life Extension. May, 2008. Consumers misled about cholesterol and statin drugs.

Polyunsaturated fatty acids and trans fatty acids in patients with the metabolic syndrome: case-control study in Korea. Lee E, Park Y, et al, *British Journal of Nutrition* (2008, Feb 28).

High omega-6 and low omega-3 fatty acids are associated with depressive symptoms and neuroticism. *Psychosom Med.* 2007 Nov 8.

Trans fat diet induces abdominal obesity and changes in insulin sensitivity in monkeys. (2007). *Obesity.*

Changes in the phenolic content of low density lipoprotein after olive oil consumption in men. (2007). *British Journal of Nutrition.*

Integrated treatment approach improves cognitive function in demented and clinically depressed patients. (2005). *Am J Alzheimer's Disease.*

Dietary fats, carbohydrate and progression of coronary atherosclerosis in postmenopausal women. www.ajcn.org/cgi/content/abstract/80/5/1175

Heimlich, Jane. (1989) *What Your Doctor Won't Tell You.*

DeCava, Judith A. Cardiovascular disease: in the news. *The Price-Pottenger Nutrition Foundation Journal.* Spring, 2008/Volume 32/Number 1.

Effects of N-3 Fatty Acids on Hepatic Triglyceride Content in Humans. Vega GL, Grundy SM, et al, *J Investig Med, 2008; 56(5): 780-785.*

Saturated fat prevents coronary artery disease? An American paradox. http://www.ajcn.org/cgi/content/full/80/5/1102.

Essential fatty acids, DHA and human brain. (2005). *Journal of Pediatrics.*

http://www.naturalnews.com/022860.html.

Fife, Bruce. (2000). *The Healing Miracle of Coconut Oil.*

Price, Weston A. (2006). *Nutrition and Physical Degeneration.*

Fallon, Sally. (2001). *Nourishing Traditions.*

Enig, Mary. (2001). *Know Your Fats.*

Omega-3 DHA and EPA for cognition, behavior and mood. (2007). Volume 12, Number 3. *Alternative Medicine Review.*

Dietary fat oxidation as a function of body fat. (2008). *American Journal of Clinical Nutrition.*

Low plasma N-3 fatty acids and dementia in older persons: the InCHIANTI study. Cherubini A, Andres-Lacueva C, et al, J Gerontol A Biol Sci Med Sci. (2007). 62(10): 1120-6.

Cod liver oil (n-3 fatty acids) as a non-steroidal anti-inflammatory drug sparing agent in rheumatoid arthritis. Galarraga B, Ho M, et al, Rheumatology. March 24 2008.

Reiser, S. (1985). Effects of dietary sugars on metabolic risk factors associated with heart disease. *Nutritional Health.*

Considerable increases in total serum cholesterol levels do not offer an explanation of the recent decline in mortality from coronary heart disease in Japan. Okayama A, Marmot MG Int J Epidemiol Dec 1993.

There is a direct association between falling cholesterol levels over the first 14 years and mortality over the following 18 years (11% overall and 14% CVD death rate increase per 1 mg/dL per year drop in cholesterol levels). Anderson KM. JAMA. 1987.

John B. Allred. Lowering serum cholesterol: who benefits? Journal of Nutrition 123: 1453-1459 (1993).

Depression of lymphocyte transformation following oral glucose ingestion. (1997). *American Journal of Clinical Nutrition.*

Role of sugars in human neutrophilic phagocytosis. (1973). American Journal of Clinical Nutrition.

Appleton, N. (1988) Lick The Sugar Habit. Fallon, Sally. Update 2003: *Soy Alert.*

Price, Weston A. (2006). *Nutrition and Physical Degeneration.*

Allan, Christian and Lutz, Wolfgang. (2000). *Life without Bread.*

New Zealand Medical Journal (Volume 113, Feb 11, 2000) Soy and the thyroid.

Blaylock, Russell L. (1997). Excitotoxins

Childhood dairy intake and adult cancer risk. (2007). American Journal of Clinical Nutrition.

Third International Symposium on the role of soy in preventing and treating chronic disease sponsored by *the American Oil Chemists' Society* in Washington, D.C. November 3, 1999.

Nutrient dietary patterns and the risk of breast and ovarian cancers. (2008). *International Journal of Cancer.*

Alcoholism: Clinical and experimental research family history of alcoholism linked to love of sweets. (2007, October 25). *Science Daily.*

Salt intake is related to soft drink consumption in children and adolescents: a link to obesity? (2008). American Journal of Clinical Nutrition.

Inconsistency between glycemic and insulemic responses to regular and fermented milk products. Am J Clin Nutr.2001;74:96–100.

High intakes of milk, but not meat, increase s-insulin and insulin resistance in 8-year-old boys. (2005) European Journal of Clinical Nutrition 59, 393–398. doi:10.1038/sj.ejcn.1602086. published online 17 November 2004.

262

Schlosser, Eric. (2001). Fast Food Nation.

Spreading the truth about soy www.soyonlineservice.co.nz.

Daniel, Kaayla. (2005). *The Whole Soy Story.*

Soda Warning? High-fructose corn syrup linked to diabetes. (2007). American Chemical Society.

Rivera, Rudy and Deutsch, Roger. (1998). Your Hidden Food Allergies Are Making You Fat.

Potential role of sugar (fructose) in the epidemic of hypertension, obesity and the metabolic syndrome, diabetes, kidney disease and cardiovascular disease. (2007). American Journal of Clinical Nutrition.

Palm and partially hydrogenated soybean oils adversely alter lipoprotein profiles compared with soybean and canola oils in moderately hyperlipidemic subjects. (2006). *American Journal of Clinical Nutrition.*

Much ado about high-fructose corn syrup in beverages: the meat of the matter. (2007). *American Journal of Clinical Nutrition.*

Intake of sugar-sweetened beverages and weight gain. (2006) *American Journal of Clinical Nutrition.*

Associations between healthy eating patterns and immune function or inflammation in overweight or obese. (2007). *American Journal of Clinical Nutrition.*

Skipping breakfast, alcohol consumption and physical inactivity as risk factors for overweight and obesity in adolescents. (2007). *European Journal of Clinical Nutrition.*

Haas, Elson (1992). *Staying Healthy with Nutrition.*

Chek, Paul. (2004). *Eat, Move and Be Healthy.*

Association of diet with serum insulin-like growth factor I in middle-aged and elderly men. (2005). *American Journal of Clinical Nutrition.*

Comparative fracture risk in vegetarians and nonvegetarians. (2007). *European Journal of Clinical Nutrition.*

Barr, S.I. and Rideout, C.A. (2004). Nutritional considerations for vegetarian athletes. *Nutrition, 20,* 696-703.

Davis, B.C. and Kris-Etherton, P.M. (2003). Achieving optimal essential fatty acid status in vegetarians: current knowledge and practical implications. Am*erican Journal of Clinical Nutrition,* 78 (supplement), 640S-646S.

Venderley, A.M. and Campbell, W.W. (2006). Vegetarian diets: Nutritional considerations for athletes. *Sports Medicine, 36, 4,* 293-305.

Deleterious effects of omitting breakfast on insulin sensitivity and fasting lipid profiles in healthy lean women. (2005). *American Journal of Clinical Nutrition.*

University of Minnesota (2007, October 15). Turn off the TV during family meals. *Science Daily.*

University of Liverpool (2007, April 25). TV food advertisements increase obese children's appetite. *Science Daily.*

Television watching increases motivated responding for food and energy intake in children. (2007). *American Journal of Clinical Nutrition.*

Plastics and Microwaves. http://www.jrussellshealth.org/microwaves.html#plastic.

The Selling of Organic. http://www.organicconsumers.org/articles/article_10652.cfm.

www.theecologist.org

Effects of overfeeding on the neuronal response to visual food cues. (2007). *American Journal of Clinical Nutrition.*

Stiegler, Petra; Cunliffe, Adam. The role of diet and exercise for the maintenance of fat-free mass and resting metabolic rate during weight loss. *Sports Medicine.* 36(3):239-262 2006.

Gaillot, M.T., et al, 2007. Self-control relies on glucose as a limited energy source: willpower is more than a metaphor. *Journal of Personality and Social Psychology*, 92 (2),325-36.

CHAPTER THREE REFERENCES

Rupp TL, Acebo C, Carskadon MA. *Chronobiol Int* 2007; 24:463-470. Evening alcohol suppresses salivary melatonin in young adults.

American College of Cardiology (2007, May 15). Heart failure patients with sleep apnea at greater risk of death, according to study. *Science Daily.*

American Academy of Sleep Medicine (2007, April 3). Sleep quantity affects morning testosterone levels in older men. *Science Daily.*

Poliquin, Charles. (2007). *BioSignature Modulation.*

Sleep loss: A novel risk factor for insulin resistance and type 2 diabetes. (2005, November). *Journal of Applied Physiology.*

Wilson, James L. (2001). *Adrenal Fatigue: The 21ˢᵗ Century Stress Syndrome.*

Environmental Health Perspectives. Volume 111. Number 7. June 2003. http://www.pubmedcentral.nih.gov.

Esther López-García, Raquel Faubel, Luz León-Muñoz, María C Zuluaga, José R Banegas and Fernando Rodríguez-Artalejo. Sleep duration, general and abdominal obesity and weight change among the older adult population of Spain. *America Journal of Clinical Nutrition.*2008 87: 310-316.

American Journal of Public Health (October 2001). (91:1671-1678).

Carnegie Mellon University (2007, October 10). Stress contributes to range of chronic diseases. Science Daily.

Coon S, Stark A, Peterson E, etal. Whole-body lietime occupational lead exposure and risk of Parkinson's disease. *Environ Health Perspect* 2006;114:1872-1876.

Shih RA, Glass TA,Bandeen-Roche K, et al. Environmental lead exposure and cognitive function in community-dwelling older adults. *Neurology* 2006;67:1556-1562.

Siblerud RI. The relationship between mercury from dental amalgam and mental health. *Am J Psychother* 1989;43:575-587.

http://www.health-science.com/microwave_hazards.html.
Effects of hostility on salivary cortisol levels in university students. Izawa S, Hirata U, et al, Shinrigaku Kenkyu, 2007; 78(3): 277-83.

Hay, Louise L. (1984). *Heal Your Body.*

Pert, Candace. (1999). *Molecules of Emotion.*

(2007). *Boulderfest.* Merrifield, Margaret. MD, CCFP.

Wilson, James L. (2001). *Adrenal Fatigue: The 21st Century Stress Syndrome.*

Schwarzbein, Diana. (2002). *The Schwarzbein Principle II.*

Shames, Richard. (2002). *Thyroid Power.*

Brownstein, David. (2007). *Iodine: Why You Need It, Why You Can't Live Without It.*

Lee, John (1999). *What Your Doctor May Not Tell You About Premenopause.*

Colditz GA. Relationship between estrogen levels, use of hormone replacement therapy and breast cancer. *J Natl Cancer Inst* 1998;90(11):814-23. 19. Thomas HV, Reeves GK, Key TJ.

Green tea catechin polyphenols attenuate behavioral and oxidative responses to intermittent hypoxia. Burckhardt IC, Gozal D, et al, Am J Respir Crit Care Med, 2008; 177(10): 1135-41.

Reiss, Uzzi. (2001). Natural Hormone Balance.

Gittleman, Ann Louise. (1998). *Before the Change.*

Poliquin, Charles. (2007). *Biosignature Modulation.*

Daniel R. Doerge, Hebron C. Chang. Inactivation of thyroid peroxidase by soy isoflavones in vitro and in vivo. *Journal of Chromatography* B Vol. 777 (1, 2); 25; September 2002: 269-79.

www.chekinstitute.com/articles

Klein RZ, Sargent JD, Larsen PR, et al. Relation of severity of maternal hypothyroidism to cognitive development of offspring. *J Med Screen* 2001;8:18-20.

Miller DW. Iodine in health and civil defense. Presented at the 24th Annual Meeting of Doctors for Disaster Preparedness in Portland, Oregon, August 6, 2006.

Guy E. Abraham, M.D.., et al, *The Original Internist*, December 2002.

L Goldemberg - La Semana Med 28:628 (1921) - cited in Wilson RH, DeEds F - The synergistic action of thyroid on fluoride toxicity. Endocrinology 26:851 (1940).

Nutrition, Hormones and Supplementation. Jerry Brainum.

(2003). *Genetic Nutrition: Hormones, Overtraining and Stress.* Dr. Eric Serrano, MD, Thomas Incledon, MS, RD.

Integrative Approach to Menopause; Tori Hudson, N.D., Norma Leslie, PhD, Holly Lucille, N.D., Sima Aidun, N.D.; June, 2004(2004).

CHAPTER FOUR REFERENCES

Poliquin, Charles. (2007). *Biosignature Modulation.*

Mayo Clinic (2008, January 4). *Moderate Exercise Yields Big Benefits.*

Associations between physical activity, body fat and insulin resistance (homeostasis model assessment) in adolescents: the European Youth Heart Study. Nico S Rizzo, Jonatan R Ruiz, Leila Oja, Tomas Veidebaum and Michael Sjöström. *American Journal of Clinical Nutrition.* 2008; 87 586-592. http://www.ajcn.org/cgi/content/abstract/87/3/586.

Combined influence of physical activity and television viewing on the risk of overweight in US youth. Eisenmann JC, Bartee RT, et al. *Int J Obese* (Lond), 2008 Jan 22.

Rhea et al., "A comparison of linear and daily undulating periodized programs with equated volume and intensity for local muscular endurance." Journal of Strength and Conditioning Research 2002; 16(2): 250-5.

Whey protein ingestion in elderly persons results in greater muscle protein accrual than ingestion of its constituent essential amino acid content. Katsanos CS, Chinkes DL, et al, Nutrition Research, 2008; 28(10): 651-8

www.chekinstitute.com/articles.

www.charlespoliquin.com/articles.

Poliquin, Charles. (1997). *The Poliquin Principles.*

Strength training and adiposity in premenopausal women: strong, healthy and empowered study. (2007). *American Journal of Clinical Nutrition* 86: 566-572.

Wiley-Blackwell (2008, January 9). Strength training of neck muscles relieves chronic pain. *Science Daily.*

Banz, William J. Effects of resistance versus aerobic training on coronary artery disease risk factors. *Experimental Biology and Medicine* 228:434-440. (2003).

Metabolic and anabolic diets for muscle mass and minimizing body fat; nutritional supplements; manipulating hormone levels to maximize the anabolic effects of training and prevent overtraining; enhance performance with supplementation. Dr. Mauro DiPasquale, MD. March, 2001.

Consumption of green tea favorably affects oxidative stress markers in weight-trained men. Panza VS, da Silva EL, et al, *Nutrition*, 2008; 24(5): 433-42.

Boirie, Y., Dangin, M., Gachon, P., Vasson, M.P., Maubois, J.L. and Beaufrere, B. (1997) Slow and fast dietary proteins differently modulate postprandial protein accretion. *Proclamations of National Academy of Sciences* 94, 14930-14935.

Boston University (2008, February 7). Weight training reduces fat and improve metabolism in mice. *Canadian Journal of Applied Physiology.*

266

Sprint interval and traditional endurance training induce similar improvements in peripheral arterial stiffness and flow mediated dilation in healthy humans. (2008, April). American Journal of Physiology.

Strength training in the elderly: effects on risk factors for age-related diseases. Hurley, Ben F.; Roth, Stephen M. Sports Medicine. 30(4):249-268, 2000.

Fat metabolism and acute resistance exercise in trained men. Michael J. Ormsbee, John P. Thyfault, Emily A. Johnson, Raymond M. Kraus, Myung Dong Choi, and Robert C. Hickner. *J Appl Physiology* 102: 1767-1772, 2007.

Effect of post-exercise supplement consumption on adaptations to resistance training. Janet Walberg Rankin, PhD. Journal of the American College of Nutrition, Vol. 23, No. 4,322-330. 2004.

Journal of Applied Physiology. Vol. 82, No. 1, pp. 298-304, January 1997. Metabolism.

Poliquin, Charles. (2007). Biosignature Modulation.

Poliquin, Charles. (1997). *The Poliquin Principles.*

John Wiley & Sons, Inc. (2006, October 7). Weight training does not increase strength but may slow progression in osteoarthritis patients. *Science Daily.*

Tarnopolsky, M.A. 2008. Sex differences in exercise metabolism and the role of 17-beta estradiol. *Medicine & Science in Sports & Exercise,* 40 (4), 648-54.

Wust, R.C.I., et al. 2008. Sex differences in contractile properties and fatigue resistance of human skeletal muscle. *Experimental Physiology.* In press.

Hunter, S.K., et al. 2004. Men are more fatigable than strength-match women when performing intermittent submaximal contractions. Journal of Applied Physiology, 96, 2125-32.

Relaxation therapy in the background of standard hypertensive drug treatment is effective in management of moderate to severe essential hypertension. Saudi Med J, 2007; 28(9): 1353-6.

Edwards L. Meditation as medicine: benefits go beyond relaxation. Advance for Nurse Practitioners. 2003;11(5):49-52.

2005. The Seven Spiritual Laws of Yoga. Deepak Chopra. David Simon.

Yoga therapy as an add-on treatment in the management of patients with schizophrenia--a randomized controlled trial. Acta Psychiatr Scand, 2007; 116(3): 226-32.

Schwarzbein, Diana. (2002). *The Schwarzbein Principle II.*

Mackinnon, L.T. (1999). *Advanced in Exercise Immunology.*

Lakier Smith, Lucille. Overtraining, excessive exercise and altered immunity. *Sports Medicine.* 33(5):347-364, 2003.

University Of Guelph (2007, June 29). Interval training burns more fat, increases fitness. Blackwell Publishing Ltd. (2006, September 18). No time to exercise is no excuse.

Wiley-Blackwell (2008, January 9). Strength training of neck muscles relieves chronic pain.

Poliquin, Charles. (2007). *Biosignature Modulation.*

www.chekinstitute.com/articles.

Page, Linda. (2004). *Healthy Healing.*

Cherkin DC, Deyo RA, Sherman KJ, et al. Characteristics of visits to licensed acupuncturists, chiropractors, massage therapists and naturopathic physicians. *Journal of the American Board of Family Practice.* 2002;15(6):463-472.

Effect of green tea on volatile sulfur compounds in mouth air. Lodhia P, Yaegaki K, et al, *J Nutr Sci Vitaminol,* 2008; 54(1): 89-94.

Koes BW, Assendelft WJ, van der Heijden GJ, et al. Spinal manipulation for low back pain. An updated systematic review of randomized clinical trials. *Spine.* 1996;21(24):2860-2871.

Effects of strength training on total and regional body composition. M. S. Treuth, A. S. Ryan, R. E. Pratley, M. A. Rubin, J. P. Miller, B. J. Nicklas, J. Sorkin, S. M. Harman, A. P. Goldberg and B. F. Hurley. *Journal of Applied Physiology,* 77:614-620, 1994.

University of Missouri-Columbia (2007, October 10). More than a pill: complementary medicine can help with chronic pain.

David W. Dunstan, PhD, Robin M. Daly, PhD, Neville Owen, PhD, Damien Jolley, MSC, Maximilian de Courten, MD, Jonathan Shaw, MD and Paul Zimmet, PhD High-intensity resistance training improves glycemic control in older patients with type 2diabetes. *Diabetes Care.* 25:1729-1736, 2002.

Imai K and Nakachi K. Cross sectional study of effects of drinking green tea on cardiovascular and liver diseases. BJM 1995; 310:693-696

CHAPTER FIVE REFERENCES

Poliquin, Charles. (2007). *BioSignature Modulation.*

Eidenier, Jr., PhD. Harry. Boenning, Daniel. (2008). *Anti-Aging Nutritional Factors.*

Metabolic and Anabolic Diets for Muscle Mass and Minimizing Body Fat; Nutritional Supplements; Manipulating Hormone Levels to Maximize the Anabolic Effects of Training and Prevent Overtraining; Enhance Performance with Supplementation. Dr. Mauro DiPasquale, MD, March, 2001.

(2007). Effects of dietary supplements on depressive symptoms in older patients. Gariballa S, Forster S. *American Journal of Clinical Nutrition.*

(2007). Dietary Supplementation and Quality of Life of Older Patients. Gabriballa S, Forster S, *Journal of American Geriatric Society.*

(2007). Usage patterns, health and nutritional status of long-term multiple dietary supplement users: a cross-sectional study. Block G, Jensen CD. *Nutrition Journal.*

(2000). *Nutrition and Supplementation: Just the Facts.* Dr. Eric Serrano, MD.

(2002). *Journal of the American Medical Association.* Suboptimal vitamin status. (287(23):3127-9).

Lipski, Elizabeth. (2000). *Digestive Wellness.*

Eidenier, Jr., PhD, Harry O. (2008). *Acid-base balance and hypochlorhydria.*

Wright, Jonathan. (2005). *Why stomach acid is good for you.*

Effects of n-3 polyunsaturated fatty acids in subjects with nonalcoholic fatty liver disease . Spadaro L, Purrello F, et al. *Digestion of Liver Disease.* December 2007.

Treatment for 2 mos with n-3 polyunsaturated fatty acids reduces adiposity and some atherogenic factors but does not improve insulin sensitivity in women with type 2 diabetes: a randomized controlled study. Kabir M, Skurnik G, et al. *American Journal of Clinical Nutrition.* (2007). 86(6): 1670-1679.

The role of an intravenous fat emulsion composed of fish oil in a parenteral nutrition-dependent patient with hypertriglyceridemia. Gura K, Puder M, *Nutr Clin Pract,* 2007; 22(6): 664-72.

Docosahexaenoic acid (DHA) supplementation in atopic eczema: a randomized, double-blind, controlled trial. Koch C, Dolle S, et al, *Br J Dermatol,* 2008; 158(4):786-92.

Docosahexaenoic acid supplementation decreases remnant-like particle-cholesterol and increases the (n-3) index in hypertriglyceridemic men. Kelley DS, Siegel D, et al, *J Nutr,* 2008; 138(1): 30-5.

Docosahexaenoic acid-rich fish oil improves heart rate variability and heart rate responses to exercise in overweight adults. Ninio DM, Hill AM, et al, *Br J Nutr,* 2008 Mar 13.

Long chain omega-3 fatty acids intake, fish consumption and mental disorders in the SUN cohort study. Sanchez-Villegas A, Henriquez P, et al, *Eur J Nutr,* 2007;46(6): 337-46.

Ohara K. Omega-3 fatty acids in mood disorders. Seishin Shinkeigaku Zasshi. 2005;107(2):118-26. *J. Nutr.* 137:2629-2634, December 2007.

(2008). Wright, Jonathan. www.wrightnewsletter.com/etips/ht200803/ht20080319b.html.

Kidd, Parris. (2007). Omega-3 DHA and EPA for cognition, behavior and mood. *Alternative Medicine Review,* Volume 12, Number 3.

Metcalf RG, James MJ, Gibson RA, et al. *Am J Clin Nutri* (2007). Effects of fish oil supplementation on myocardial fatty acids in humans.

Child & Family Research Institute (2008, March 11). Typical North American diet is deficient in omega-3 fatty acids. *Science Daily.*

Poliquin, Charles. (2007). *BioSignature Modulation.*

Dose-dependent effects of docosahexaenoic acid-rich fish oil on erythrocyte docosahexaenoic acid and blood lipid levels. Milte CM, Coates AM, et al, *British Journal of Nutrition.* Oct 2007; 1-6.

Omega-3 Fatty acid supplementation and regular moderate exercise: differential effects of a combined intervention on neutrophil function. Hill AM, Worthley C, et al, *Br J Nutr,* 2007; 98(2): 300-9.

Low plasma N-3 fatty acids and dementia in older persons: the InCHIANTI study. Cherubini A, Andres-Lacueva C, et al, *J Gerontol A Biol Sci Med Sci.* (2007). 62(10): 1120-6.

Essential n-3 fatty acids in pregnant women and early visual acuity maturation in term infants. Innis SM, Friesen RW, et al. *Am J Clin Nutr*. (2008). 87(3): 548-57.

Cod liver oil (n-3 fatty acids) as a non-steroidal anti-inflammatory drug sparing agent in rheumatoid arthritis. Galarraga B, Ho M, et al, *Rheumatology*. March 24 2008.

Multivitamin supplementation improves nutritional status and bone quality in aged care residents. Grieger JA, Nowson CA. *Eur J Clin Nutr*. 2007 Nov 28.

Hollis BW, Wagner CL. Assessment of dietary vitamin D requirements during pregnancy and lactation. *American Journal of Clinical Nutrition*. (2004). 79:717-726.

Garland, CG, Grant WB, Mohr SB. What is the dose-response relationship between vitamin D and cancer risk? *Nutrition Review*. 2007; 65:S91-S95.

Use of multivitamins, intake of B vitamins and risk of ovulatory infertility. Chavarro JE, Willett WC. *Fertil Steril*. 2008; 89(3): 668-76.

Effect of vitamin C supplementation on lipid peroxidation, muscle damage and inflammation after 30-min exercise at 75% v.o.2max. Nakhostin-Roohi B, Babaei P, et al, *J Sports Med Phys Fitness*, 2008; 48(2): 217-24.

Effects of multivitamin supplementation on DNA damage in lymphocytes from elderly volunteers. Ribeiro ML, Arcari DP, et al, *Mech Ageing Dev*. 2007 Aug 15.

Safety of vitamin D3 in adults with multiple sclerosis. Kimball SM, Ursell MR, et al. *Am J Clin Nutr*. 2007; 86(3): 645-51.

Vitamin D deficiency in elderly men. Bouuaert C, Vanmeerbeek M, et al, *Presse Med*, 2008; 37(2 Pt 1): 191-200.

Serum vitamin D and subsequent occurrence of type 2 diabetes," Knekt P, Laaksonen M, et al, Epidemiol, 2008; 19(5): 666-71.

Prevalence of vitamin D insufficiency in obese children and adolescents. Smotkin-Tangorra M, Purushothaman R. *Journal of Pediatric Endocrinology and Metabolism*. 2007; 20(7): 817-823.

Vitamin D supplementation and total mortality: a meta-analysis of randomized controlled trials. Autier P, Gandini S, *Archives of Internal Medicine*. 2007; 167(16): 1730-7.

Higher serum vitamin D concentrations are associated with longer leukocyte telomere length in women. Richards JB, Valdes AM, et al. *Am J Clin Nutr*. 2007; 86(5): 1420-1425. Dietary vitamin D and calcium intake and premenopausal breast cancer risk in a German case-control study. Abbas S, Linseisen J, Chang-Claude *J. Nutr Cancer*. 2007; 59(1): 54-61.

Hicks GE et al. Associations between vitamin D status and pain in older adults: The Invecchiare in Chianti Study. *J Am Geriatric Soc* 2008 May; 56:785.

Tsitouras PD, Bucciardo F, Salbe AD, Hweard C, Harman SM. High Omega-3 Fat Intake Improves Insulin Sensitivity and Reduces DRP and IL6, but does not Affect Other Endocrine Axes in Older Adults. *Horm Metab Res*. 2008 Mar;40(3):199-205.

Haas, Elson (1992). *Staying Healthy with Nutrition*.

Pain, March 2000. Martin Tramer, et al., University Hospital, Geneva.

270

Eidenier, Jr., PhD. Harry, Boenning, Daniel. (2008). *Anti-Aging Nutritional Factors.*

Beausoleil M, Weiss K, et al, *Can J Gastroenterol,* 2007; 21(11): 732-6. (2008). *American Journal of Clinical Nutrition.* www.ajcn.org/cgi/content/abstract/87/3/534.

The New York Time. Fat factors.The effect of probiotics on gut flora, level of endotoxin and child-Pugh score in cirrhotic patients. Lata J, Novotny I. (2006). *Eur J Gastroenterol Hepatol,* 2007; 19(12): 1111-3.

Yogurt containing probiotic lactobacillus rhamnosus GR-1 and L. reuteri RC-14 Helps resolve moderate diarrhea and increases CD4 count in HIV/AIDS patients. Anukam C, Osazuma EO, et al, *J Clin Gastroenterol,* 2008; 42(3): 239-243.

Lipski, Elizabeth. (2000). *Digestive Wellness.*

The effect of probiotics on Helicobacter pylori eradication. Park SK, Park DI, et al, *Hepatogastroenterology,* 2007; 54(79): 2032-6.

Page, Linda. (2004). *Healthy Healing.*

Jeavons HS. Prevention and treatment of vulvovaginal candidiasis using exogenous lactobacillus. *J Obstet Gynecol Neonatal Nurse.* 2003 May-Jun;32(3):287-96.

Long-term effect of magnesium consumption on the risk of symptomatic gallstone disease among men. Tsai CJ, Leitzmann MF, et al, *Am J Gastroenterol.* 2007 Dec 12.

Stadlbauer V, Mookerjee RP, Hodges S, Wright GAK, Davies NA, Jalan R. Effect of probiotic treatment on deranged neutrophil function and cytokine responses in patients with compensated alcoholic cirrhosis. Journal of Hepatology. (Elsevier) 25 March 2008.

(2005). Survival Medicine for the 21st Century. Mark Sircus.

University of Maryland Medical Center, Center for Integrative Medicine, Alternative Complementary Medicine Supplements database. www.umm.edu/altmed/ConsLookups/Supplements.html.

Role of magnesium sulfate in postoperative pain management for patients undergoing thoracotomy. Ozcan PE, Tugrul S, et al, *J Cardiothorac Vasc Anesth,* 2007; 21(6): 827-31.

Jee SH, Miller ER, Guallar E, et al. The effect of magnesium supplementation on blood pressure: a meta-analysis of randomized clinical trials. *Am J Hypertension.* 2002. Aug;15(8):691-6.

Magnesium intake and risk of type 2 diabetes: a meta-analysis. Larsson SC, Wolk A, J Intern Med, 2007; 262(2): 208-14.

Aikawa LK, Magnesium: Its Biological Significance, CRC Press, Boca Raton, Fl, 1981.

Michael Murray, N.D. and Joseph Pizzorno, N.D. (1998). Encyclopedia of Natural Medicine.

Bolton JL, Pisha E, Zhang F, et al. Role of quinoids in estrogen carcinogenesis. Chem Res Toxicol 1998;11:1113-27.

Magnesium, calcium, potassium and sodium intakes and risk of stroke in male smokers. Larsson SC, Virtanen MJ, et al, Arch Intern Med, 2008; 168(5); 459-65. http://ods.od.nih.gov/factsheets/magnesium.asp. Accessed February 28, 2008.

Appel LJ. Nonpharmacologic therapies that reduce blood pressure: A fresh perspective. Clin Cardiol 1999;22:1111-5.

Haas, Elson (1992). Staying Healthy with Nutrition.

Sircus, Mark. (2008). Winning the War on Cancer.

USDA/Agricultural Research Service (2004, May 10). Lack Energy? Maybe It's Your Magnesium Level.

ABOUT THE AUTHOR

Paula has helped people with hormonal imbalances, food cravings, depression, cancer, diabetes, digestive distress and many other health complaints for over twenty years. She is a highly sought-after expert for nutrition, exercise and lifestyle transformation. Paula holds a Masters degree in Holistic Nutrition, a Bachelors degree in Kinesiology and numerous professional health and fitness certifications. She is known for producing results *naturally*. Paula is a national seminar presenter and keynote speaker as well as a health, nutrition and fitness columnist. Paula resides in Phoenix, Arizona with her Rottweiler, Teddy Bear.

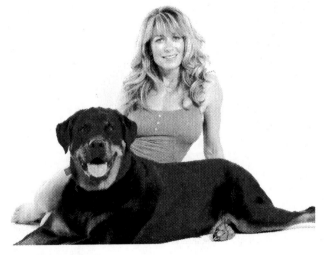

Contact information

Website: www.PaulaOwens.com

Blog: http://thepowerof4-paula.blogspot.com